Caring for the Older Adult

Lynn Basford

Karran Thorpe

Published in 2004 by:
Nelson Thornes Ltd
Delta Place
27 Bath Road
CHELTENHAM
GL53 7TH
United Kingdom

04 05 06 07 08/ 10 9 8 7 6 5 4 3 2 1

A catalogue record for this book is available from the British Library

ISBN 0 7487 8524 8

Page make-up by Acorn Bookwork Ltd

Printed in Great Britain by Ashford Colour Press

The publishers would like to thank Emap Healthcare Open Learning and Richard Smith for permission to reproduce photographs

Contents

INTRODUCTION

Demographic trends as well as changes in health and social care policy have major implications for the care of older people, no matter where that care is delivered or which professionals deliver it. Care of older people is now at the top of the agenda for health-care educators, professionals, scientists and government.

AIMS OF THIS BOOK

This book aims to help you explore what it means to develop your professional practice to enhance the quality of care you and your team members provide to older people. It encourages you to do five things:

- Consider the demands and responsibilities that you have as an active, lifelong learner and health-care professional.
- Consider the demands and responsibilities of your central role in providing quality care for older people.
- Understand your personal responsibility for developing your professional skills and knowledge.
- Evaluate and challenge your personal and professional values, attitudes and beliefs about good practice with older people.
- Gain a profile of research, management, and professional skills and knowledge. This perspective will be unique to you and your personal requirements, yet it will give you enhanced insights into the work of your colleagues in the multidisciplinary team in your setting.

The eight learning outcomes will help you enhance your work with older people, to:

- Appreciate and value yourself fully as a health-care professional working with older people.
- Empathize with older people as individuals, acknowledging their uniqueness.
- Recognize older people as central to your care.
- Consider new perspectives about your role as a health-care professional caring for older people.
- Develop new approaches, where appropriate, to your day-to-day practice with older people.
- Participate fully in improving the quality of care for older people.
- Improve your ability to appraise and evaluate the care you and your colleagues provide to older people (i.e. enhance your critical-thinking skills).
- Develop your skills in reflexive practice.

All the chapters are organized in a similar way:

- Objectives
- Introduction
- Activities scattered throughout
- Summary
- Key points
- References
- Further reading (in some chapters).

'OLDER PEOPLE': A WORD ABOUT LANGUAGE

Throughout this book we have chosen, primarily, to use the term 'older people', although you may prefer other terms, such as patient, client, resident, and service user. If you prefer another term, you can simply use it as you work through the book. Another editorial choice was to use a person's first name where possible, rather than the more formal Mr, Mrs, Miss or Ms followed by their surname. Enhancing respect and dignity are critical in all interactions with others, older people as well as colleagues. In practice it is essential to ask people how they would like to be addressed, by first name or surname. Regardless of the typical practice in your work setting, always respect the person's preference.

ORGANIZING YOUR LEARNING AS HEALTH-CARE PROFESSIONALS

1

OBJECTIVES

- Describe the essential components of problem-based learning.
- Begin the process of problem-based learning by working through the activities in this chapter.
- Describe four learning styles.
- Define critical thinking.
- Describe five elements of critical thinking.
- Explain a three-stage model of reflective learning.
- Identify and describe the purpose and main elements of a learning plan.
- Explain the key features of a reflective learning journal.
- Identify the key elements in a professional and personal portfolio.

INTRODUCTION

Around the world, the population is ageing. Therefore we need to look at health issues related specifically to older people, and we also need to consider the implications for the rest of the population. For instance, the advent of older mothers creates new issues in midwifery. This chapter stimulates you to think for yourself about the challenges associated with caring for older people. Its goal is to encourage your thoughtful, critical reflection on the information you read and your exploration of the possibilities that you imagine may promote quality care for all older people. Figure 1.1 shows how family support promotes the health and well-being of older people.

This chapter introduces several important concepts that will support you in your learning: problem-based learning, learning style, critical thinking and reflective learning. It offers several strategies to help you understand how you might demonstrate your learning; for example, it includes descriptions of learning plans, reflective learning journals and professional portfolios. It introduces the case study contained in the appendix. The case study will help you learn about these important concepts. It illustrates the relationship between information provided in a case study and the opportunities for learning what you need to know to care for older people.

The chapter primarily focuses on you, the learner, by providing a review of essential skills (i.e. critical thinking and reflexive skills) and strategies (i.e. learning plans, reflective learning journals and portfolios). You are encouraged to enhance your skills by working through the study activities and using the strategies described in this chapter. These skills are essential to becoming a self-directed learner ready for lifelong

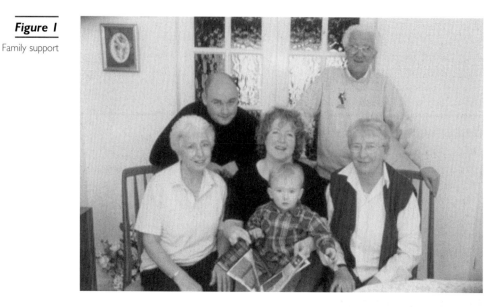

Figure 1

Family support

learning. When you actively engage in the learning process, you reap benefits of personal and professional growth. As a health-care professional, you are best positioned to apply your knowledge, skills and attitudes to the older people within your care.

PROBLEM-BASED LEARNING

Learning is an active and demanding process. Successful learners invest time, energy and commitment in their learning activities. A popular approach to learning, called problem-based learning (P-BL), context-based learning or inquiry-based learning, accommodates several essential characteristics – problem-oriented, student-centred and small groups – as identified by Rideout and Carpio (2001). Boud (1985) suggests: 'the principal idea behind problem-based learning is that *the starting point for learning should be a problem*, a query, or a puzzle that the learner wishes to solve' (p. 13, original emphasis). The second characteristic emphasizes the student-centred nature of this approach, hence the need to be a self-directed learner (S-DL). This characteristic speaks directly to students about the personal nature of the learning process. Typically, P-BL employs a problem from a real-world situation and uses that problem to stimulate the learning process.

Working in small groups, the third characteristic, and with a brief scenario about a particular problem or case study, students word-storm to determine the knowledge they need to understand the situation. They develop objectives to address the gaps between their current knowledge and what they need to explore to resolve the case study. Each student accepts responsibility for acquiring the appropriate information to address a specific objective. In the subsequent tutorial session, students report their findings and ask each other questions to ensure that each student understands the information presented. Additional segments of the case study are provided as students request. The process of word-storming, questioning, objective setting and information sharing continues until students determine that they have explored all avenues appropriate to resolving the problem.

The P-BL approach to learning places responsibility with each learner and relates to the need for specific skills in learning. Significantly, the P-BL approach supports students in 'learning how to learn', thereby enhancing students to accept the principles of lifelong learning. Thus, students are best prepared to function competently and confidently in a constantly changing health-care arena. Simultaneously, students learn how to work well together as members of a group sharing common goals. To that end, students engage regularly in evaluation of the group process as well as self-evaluation and peer evaluation. With this overview of P-BL, it is appropriate to consider the problem in some detail as well as an example to illustrate how this process is operationalized.

DEFINING A PROBLEM

A problem, or case study, is the description of an individual, family, group or community that focuses on specific issues requiring the assistance of health-care professionals. Problems, reflecting real-life situations, are typically written in one to four scenarios. Each scenario is intended to stimulate discussion of the problem, and the information is presented in a sequential manner. For instance, the second scenario will provide information to support the direction of inquiry, which essentially may answer initial questions or hypotheses identified by students during the first word-storming session. Or the second scenario may eliminate some of the avenues pursued in the first scenario, which directs students in their learning. Appropriate clinical data may also accompany the scenario information. The scenario and the clinical data are provided to students in a timely fashion, as requested or appropriate, but only after each scenario is fully explored.

Importantly, the tutor has a set of key concepts and learning objectives specific to each problem. With this information the tutor guides the students as they explore the learning possibilities in each scenario. The tutor's role is not to provide the answers but to facilitate student-directed learning. Over a short period of time, students resolve the problem and are prepared to examine another problem that describes another real-life situation.

This book gives you an opportunity to learn about the P-BL approach by exploring the case study of Mary.

CASE STUDY OF MARY

Mary is 70 years old. Her husband, who was in the army, died several years ago. At one time, his army work meant frequent moves to different localities. Mary has lived in 30 different houses during her lifetime, and she has lived in her present council house for 20 years. She has six children, three sons and three daughters. Her sons are married with families and live outside London. Her youngest daughter (aged 36 years) is Heather. Heather and her husband, Ron, and their children, Emily (aged 10 years) and Tommy (aged 4 years), live with Mary in her house in London. Mary's eldest daughter, Sandra, lives with her family on the other side of London. Her middle daughter, Caroline, lives with her family in the Midlands. Table 1.1 shows Mary's medical history.

Table 1.1

Mary's medical history

1989	Heart operation for an aneurysm
1993	Broken leg
Nov 1996	Fall; discharged from accident and emergency
Nov/Dec 1996	Hip replacement operation
Dec 1996	Suspected clot on lung, and pneumonia
Dec 1996	Deep-vein thrombosis
Mar 1997	Referral to day hospital

Mary's comments

Heather goes out to work. She has two children. Whoever gets in first does the cooking. It's usually me four days a week. Sometimes you can get the children to help but the four-year-old, well, he's just an ordinary four-year-old. We've got three rooms downstairs, the lounge and the dining room leading to the kitchen, and a small toilet. Upstairs there are the bedrooms and the bathroom.

Heather's comments

I was 16 when we moved here and then I met my husband and we decided to stay here because I didn't like to leave Mum on her own, although she was much younger then. It is nice; I mean, I wouldn't dream of going now, especially now Mum's not well. I'm quite happy to stay here and the children are happy here. I mean, if we were to move, if we were to be rehoused by the council, we'd probably get a flat and at the moment, we've got a nice garden, a nice big house, the children have each got a bedroom; it's fine for us. They would have to move Mum as well and I think she'd be very, very unhappy if she had to move. She's always said, 'I wouldn't mind living by myself.' But she doesn't want to move. I know that. Am I a carer? I'm just the daughter, I've never classed myself as a carer before.

Activity

In a P-BL tutorial situation there would be a group of 12 students and a tutor to consider the information provided in this first scenario. However, you may also work through the steps on your own:

- Summarize what you know about Mary's situation.
- What evidence do you have to support the facts you summarized?

- Identify at least three facts that you need to know before you can respond to this scenario.
- Briefly describe how you will find the answers to the need-to-know facts that you identified in the previous item.
- Write one objective you could pursue to learn more about Mary's situation.

Learning is enhanced to the degree that students employ skills associated with learning styles, sound critical thinking and reflective learning. Each of these topics is discussed in turn.

LEARNING STYLE

Kolb (1984) presents a four-stage theory of learning that supports effect and experience in concert with cognition and reflection. Essentially, students progress through a cycle of learning that commences with a 'concrete experience' upon which they reflect and form abstractions. Later on, students use the knowledge gained from this experience in testing the implications for other situations. Over time, these instances of learning accumulate and contribute to the sequential learning process. Kolb describes four styles of learning:

- **Accommodator**: impulsive but adaptable, they are personally involved in situations and prefer change rather than routine.
- **Assimilator**: logical and perceptual, they organize and synthesize information, create models and test theories.
- **Diverger**: feeling and observing, they listen with an open mind when collecting information.
- **Converger**: symbolic and practical, they apply theories and ideas in problem solving.

Kolb explains that individuals tend to have a favourite or dominant learning style. However, individuals also have the capacity to expand their preferential styles to incorporate other styles of learning. Here again we see the idea of active learning.

Loo (1997) examines the utility of Kolb's (1984) experiential learning model and learning style inventory of 1985 (LSI-1985) among 172 undergraduate students in four different management courses. Regardless of the course, one objective was to support students to explore personal discovery and growth. Unfortunately, one finding was that 'about 39% of the students reported that they have not thought about ways to improve their own learning effectiveness' (Loo, 1997, p. 49). This finding emphasizes the need to think about one's learning style and to seriously contemplate how one might develop new approaches to learning. Loo reports that students found the exercise 'interesting and personally useful' (*ibid.*, p. 49) even though approximately half of the students maintained their same learning style from the first to the second administration of the LSI-1985. Nevertheless, through reflection and self-appraisal, students may learn to develop other styles of learning. Awareness of the different learning styles enables students to pursue self-directed learning (S-DL) with increased confidence. One benefit of being able to employ different learning styles is that students can then use the best learning style to suit the situation.

Rakoczy and Money (1995) investigated 'the learning style of nursing students over the 3 years of a diploma program' (p. 171). The cohort included 176 female nursing students in year 1, 138 in year 2, and 144 in year 3. They discovered little variation from year 1 to year 3 and 'when the mean scores for years 1, 2, and 3 were plotted on the grid the dominant learning style was that of assimilator which combines the learning steps of AC "thinking" and RO "watching"' (Rakoczy and Money, 1995, p. 172). Given the complexity inherent in a changing society, Rakoczy and Money suggest that nurses and, by extension, other health-care professionals would be well served in developing both convergent and divergent skills. Hence they conclude that educators who provide a balance of learning styles support professionals to prepare for a changing work environment. Thompson and Crutchlow (1993), in their review of the literature on learning styles, conclude:

> *Ultimately, the goal of nursing education should be to provide students with the skills for lifelong learning. Such skills include the ability to view problems in a variety of ways, the ability to gather appropriate information to solve them, and the ability to generate alternate solutions. Thus, educators must strive to challenge students beyond their present capabilities by exposing them to new ways of learning. (p. 39)*

Activity

- Obtain at least one reference regarding learning styles. Briefly describe what you have learned about learning styles that helps you to understand how you learn.
- Refer to the case study on Mary. Consider each of the four learning styles and identify what you know about Mary. That is, if your primary learning style were accommodator, what would you say about Mary? Repeat this process for each of the learning styles.
- Identify one objective that would help you to expand your learning styles. For instance, consider the one style that you would currently find difficult and explore how you might develop strengths in that learning style.

CRITICAL THINKING AND SKILLS TO ENHANCE LEARNING

Critical thinking is frequently explored by researchers and educators. Nevertheless, despite considerable attention, critical thinking remains elusive in its definition and application, as do the strategies that enhance or hinder its development. Currently there are only a few discipline-specific models and approaches to critical thinking, e.g. Facione and Facione (1996), Kataoka-Yahiro and Saylor (1994) and Miller and Malcolm (1990). Consequently, to date, most researchers present their perceptions about the unique and essential features of critical thinking that apply across disciplines. Watson and Glaser (1980, 1994) are leaders in this field. Although numerous definitions exist, Watson and Glaser (1994) define critical thinking in terms of attitudes, knowledge, and skills:

> *(1) attitudes of inquiry that involve an ability to recognize the existence of problems and an acceptance of the general need for evidence in support of what is asserted to be true; (2) knowledge of the nature of valid inferences, abstractions, and generalizations in which the weight or accuracy of different kinds of evidence are logically determined; and (3) skills in employing and applying the above attitudes and knowledge. (p. 9)*

In health-care arenas, competence, a concept related to critical thinking, is defined in terms of knowledge, skills, understanding and experience (Basford, 2003). In responding to the debate about how well nurses were prepared to practise competently on entering their professional roles, the United Kingdom Central Council (UKCC, 2001) recommends a serious review of educational programming. Basford presents an outcomes-competence model that addresses practice and technical outcomes and competencies. She reports:

> *To achieve total competence the student is required to demonstrate the knowledge, skill and understanding of each component of clinical practice that develops into a comprehensive portfolio. ... Assessment would be by a collection of evidence contained within a portfolio of learning, demonstrating competence through clinical and academic achievement. (p. 481)*

Accordingly, she concludes that nurses, and all health-care professionals, need to develop a range of competencies for practice in any care setting. Hence critical thinking is an essential component that enhances safe, ethical and competent care, which all health-care professionals need to employ in their daily practice.

In 1994 Watson and Glaser introduced a new version of their earlier tools to assess critical thinking. Form S of the Watson and Glaser Critical Thinking Appraisal (Watson and Glaser, 1994) is a 40-item tool that accommodates the theoretical concept of critical thinking. Here are its five subtests (Watson and Glaser, 1994, pp. 9–10):

1 **Inference**: discriminating among degrees of truth of inferences drawn from given data.

2   **Recognition of assumptions**: recognizing unstated assumptions or presuppositions in given statements or assertions.

3   **Interpretations**: weighing evidence and deciding if generalizations based on the given data are warranted.

4   **Deductions**: determining whether certain conclusions necessarily follow from information in given statements or premises.

5   **Evaluation of arguments**: distinguishing between arguments that are strong and relevant and those that are weak or irrelevant to a particular issue.

Loo and Thorpe (1999) describe the psychometric properties of Form S. It is the composite of the five subtests that provides a score on critical thinking. Individually, each subtest is insufficient to provide an indicator of critical thinking. Loo and Thorpe offer two major conclusions:

> *The new Form S needs further psychometric refinements before it can be confidently used in place of the longer Forms A and B. ... Form S has shown itself to be free from gender or faculty effects in this study and demonstrated its usefulness as a teaching tool and means of stimulating reflective learning about critical thinking. (p. 1002)*

Although not specifically developed for use by any one discipline, this appraisal of critical thinking emphasizes the significance of the sophisticated nature of thinking that is required among health-care professionals. When health-care professionals employ sound critical-thinking skills, they are in the best position to judge the evidence in the literature on clinical practice and to determine the application of new strategies in clinical practice.

Staib (2003, p. 498) notes that the National League for Nursing Accrediting Commission (2002, p. 3) stipulates that nurse graduates are expected to 'demonstrate critical thinking, reflection, and problem-solving skills'. However, as Valiga (2003) states, 'many research studies report that students do not achieve the higher levels of critical thinking and cognitive development required for practice in the ambiguous, unpredictable health care arena' (p. 479). The inconsistent reporting of findings regarding growth, or lack thereof, in the development of critical-thinking skills among nursing students suggests that attention should be given to considering alternative approaches to teaching critical-thinking skills (e.g. Duchscher, 2003; Myrick and Yonge, 2004). For instance, Ironside (2003) suggests narrative pedagogy as an alternative approach to foster teaching and learning about the processes of thinking. Myrick and Yonge emphasize that the relational process established between the preceptor and the graduate student was a major determinant in the enhancement of critical-thinking ability. They conclude that 'specific preceptor behaviours are pivotal to the enhancement of critical thinking of graduate nursing students and ultimately impact on the success or failure of the preceptorship experience' (Myrick and Yonge, 2004, pp. 378–379). Finally,

Diekelmann (2003), among others, recommends thinking-in-action journals as one way for learners to enhance their reflective thinking.

Activity

Despite the confusion over definitions and measurement of critical thinking, this concept is recognized as a basic requirement for professional practice in all health-care disciplines.

- What does critical thinking mean to you?
- Obtain a copy of one of the references cited in the discussion on critical thinking and identify the main points that you learned from reading this article.
- Referring to the case study of Mary on page 3, describe three critical-thinking strategies that you can implement to gain insights into Mary's current situation.
- What is the relationship between the concepts of critical thinking, problem solving and decision making?

REFLECTIVE LEARNING

Learning is the acquisition of knowledge and real learning is demonstrated when individuals apply that knowledge to practice. Most students are familiar with didactic approaches to learning; that is, they expect to be passive recipients of information that teachers share through the lecture format. This approach accepts the teacher as an expert who determines what is to be learned and how that learning is to be assessed. P-BL espouses student-centred learning whereby students exercise control over their learning needs, objectives and activities. This approach ensures active engagement of learners who are empowered to realize meaningful learning outcomes that continually expand their individual knowledge bases. Adopting this perspective on learning how to learn is essential for realizing the responsibilities associated with lifelong learning. The notion of learning organizations entails a need to proactively identify and implement appropriate learning strategies to meet expectations of a challenging society (e.g. Senge, 1990).

Boyd and Fales (1983) define reflective learning as 'the process of internally examining and exploring an issue of concern, triggered by an experience, which creates and clarifies meaning in terms of self, and which results in a changed conceptual perspective' (p. 100). Interestingly, nine counsellors reported that they had not thought about reflection before participating in the Boyd and Fales research. However, 'once individuals became more aware of their spontaneous reflective activity and its importance to them, they expressed interest in whether they could control their own process' (*ibid.*, p. 113). Boyd and Fales conclude that reflective learning 'is a natural process used spontaneously by many people. Once aware of their own process, people spontaneously gain greater conscious control over it and seek guidance for even more effective use of it' (*ibid.*, p. 114). Many writers address the importance of reflective learning and discuss strategies to support the development of reflective thinkers, particularly in nursing and education, such as Hyrkäs *et al.* (2001), Liimatainen *et al.* (2001) and Lyons (1999).

Atkins and Murphy (1993) identify and describe three stages of the reflective process as awareness, critical analysis and new perspective. Scanlon and Chernomas (1997) describe the application of this model to nursing education. Awareness results when an individual acknowledges a discomfort or a lack of information in explaining something. It also results when individuals perceive an excitement or curiosity to learn more about a specific topic. This first stage is essential if reflection is to occur. The second stage is critical analysis, which relates directly to the elements of critical thinking described earlier. Individuals contemplate their current knowledge while thinking about the concept, situation or event or the need for knowledge and the potential application of new information. Atkins and Murphy (1993) note that this stage requires the application of many skills, such as 'self-awareness, description, critical analysis, synthesis, and evaluation' (p. 1190).

The final stage, new perspective, indicates the outcome of the analysis or the application of new information. It provides evidence that the individual has a greater understanding of the concept, situation or event. Reflection therefore stimulates change in the affective, cognitive and perhaps behavioural realms. Importantly, learning occurs regardless of the effect of these changes. For a health-care professional's practice, reflection affords an informed position that enhances the problem-solving and decision-making processes and ultimately the care provided to older people.

Wong *et al.* (1997) 'explore how teaching and learning strategies could be arranged to maximize reflective learning among post-registration nurses' (p. 478). They make a significant contribution to the literature by distinguishing between three levels of reflection:

> *Nonreflectors were those who did not demonstrate a deliberate appraisal of the issue at their disposal. These students tended to remain within their pre-existing frame of reference. The reflectors demonstrated effort in analyzing, discriminating, and evaluating various points of view, and there was evidence of arrival at insight. Critical reflectors tended to reach a level where they could redefine their original problem and redirect action to reach a transformation of perspective.* (ibid., p. 478)

Later Kember *et al.* (1999) expand the essence of these three levels of reflection. Non-reflective action includes habitual action (i.e. learned action that becomes automatic practice), thoughtful action (i.e. the use of existing knowledge without appraising the knowledge), and introspection (i.e. feelings or thoughts about oneself). Acknowledging what constitutes non-reflection supports the recognition of reflection. Reflective action entails content reflection (concerned with what), process (concerned with how) and premise (concerned with why). Content reflection and process reflection are deemed to be at the same level, whereas premise reflection is thought to be at a higher level (Kember *et al.*, 1999). Kember *et al.* explain that premise reflection 'requires a critical review of presuppositions from conscious and unconscious prior learning and their consequences'. They concluded that 'premise reflection was unlikely to be observed frequently within student journals. For writing to be coded as premise reflection, there needed to be evidence of significant change in perspective' (*ibid.*, pp. 23–24).

Together, the three stages of reflection – awareness, critical reflection and new perspective – and the three levels of reflection – non-reflectors, reflectors and critical reflectors – provide insights into the expectations about reflective learning journals. This information provides useful information for students and educators who wish to gain the most benefit from this learning strategy.

Rolfe (2003) extends the discussion of reflection to encompass reflective practice: 'In nursing, we use the term "reflective practice" to refer to the *application* of this reflective tool to an exploration of our thoughts, feelings and beliefs about our own practice' (p. 483, original emphasis). To benefit most from this activity of reflection, Pierson (1998) explains the differences between calculative and contemplative thinking. For example, Pierson suggests that calculative thinking simply results in a listing of daily activities, whereas contemplative thinking uses an interactive, conversational style of writing or communicating to develop self-awareness and understanding. Calculative thinking may be commonplace, but contemplative thinking is required in reflective practice. According to Rolfe, reflective practice supports the critical appraisal of research-based theory and knowledge and also the exploration of personal knowledge. Furthermore, reflective practice leads to reflexive practice when health-care professionals reflect *in* the clinical setting rather than simply *on* past actions. Reflection-in-action, as described by Schön (1983), indicates the standard of expert practice within any professional discipline.

Activity

- From the literature, select one theory that explains the process of reflection. Describe the central components of this theory and relate this theory to your practice as a health-care professional.
- Describe one example of reflexivity from your practice with older people.
- Identify and briefly describe three advantages and three disadvantages of reflection. You may wish to select one or two articles from the literature to support your work in this activity.
- Explain the differences between reflection *in* practice and reflection *on* practice.
- Explore the notion that effective reflection is linked to the provision of quality care to older people.

DEMONSTRATING YOUR LEARNING

There are many ways of demonstrating your learning. For instance, your learning can be demonstrated, and easily assessed, through learning plans or contracts, reflective learning journals, and professional portfolios or profiles. These learning strategies are also effective in guiding you through the learning process. As a self-directed learner, and in consultation with your tutor or counsellor, you are in the best position to identify your learning needs. Therefore, considering the important concepts of learning presented in this chapter and your interest in learning about the care of older people, you may wish to select from these strategies to demonstrate your learning.

You need to provide evidence of your learning for your tutor to evaluate. It is also important for you to adopt the practice of self-assessment or self-evaluation, consistent with the principles of P-BL and reflective learning. In P-BL tutorial sessions, students regularly participate in formative and summative evaluation processes, focusing on group process, knowledge development, attitudes, critical thinking, self-directed learning, and performance of self, other colleagues and the tutor. Constructive evaluation includes the identification of strengths and areas for improvement. Self-assessment is directly related to taking responsibility for your own learning; indeed it tends to increase communication between student and tutor and reduce anxiety associated with the evaluation process. Lyons (1999) and Jasper (1999) concur that reflective journal writing facilitates students in achieving personal development. Specifically, Jasper (1999) explains that reflective writing 'is seen as an immensely personal, and relatively safe, way of admitting strengths and weaknesses and developing as a result of dealing with these' (p. 461).

LEARNING PLANS

A learning plan, or contract, is a strategy that supports students in developing and demonstrating S-DL skills. Learning plans are simply written agreements between students and their tutors that afford structure and direction for learning activities. Knowles (1974) proposes the use of learning plans to individualize the learning needs of students. A learning plan or contract includes goals (e.g. encompassing knowledge, skills and attitudes), objectives related to the learning domains (cognitive, psychomotor and affective), learning resources and strategies, evidence of accomplishment, criteria and means of validating evidence, as well as the deadline for completing specific objectives (Crooks *et al.*, 2001; Knowles, 1974).

When learning plans are used within courses, such as completing this book, the goals and objectives need to be consistent with the book or course objectives. However, in clinical placements or experiences, learning plans provide a blueprint for individual learning identified by students. Therefore students are encouraged to demonstrate self-directedness and to gain competence and confidence by identifying a unique learning plan to capture their own learning needs within a chosen clinical setting. Often students require support in writing clear objectives, identifying objectives that are manageable, accessing resources and specifying criteria for evaluation of evidence. Remember that students retain control over their learning plans and that learning plans remain

Table 1.2 Example of a learning plan

| Name of student | | | | |
| Clinical area | | | | Date |
Learning goals	**Learning objectives**	**Learning resources and strategies**	**Evidence**	**Criteria for evaluation and date of completion**
To develop knowledge about communicating with older people	To identify and describe three key elements in the interview process	Texts and other references in the library, specific to communication and interviews	Six-page paper describing three principles of effective interviewing and application of those principles in interviewing older people	Paper will be marked by tutor using the following criteria: clarity, coherence, comprehensiveness, and logical development of ideas Worth 25% Due 1 February 2005
To develop communication skills specific to older people	To develop skills in communicating with older people by using the concepts and principles of communication theory (listening, questioning, etc.)	Texts and other references in the library, specific to communication Tutor Discuss key concepts with nurse manager Interview two individuals who are not related and are in different age groups	Reflective learning journal about three communication skills that you are developing and how theory relates to practice	Reflective learning journal will be marked by tutor using the following criteria: clear identification of skills, insights into need to change some habitual practices, and progress on developing effective interviewing skills Worth 15% Due 1 March 2005
			Brief synopsis of two interviews, indicating three principles of communication and what you learned from the interviewees	The brief synopsis will be evaluated by your tutor using the following criteria: clarity, comprehensiveness, and logical development of principles and application of same Due 1 April 2005
To demonstrate an attitude of inquiry into the communication needs of older people	To identify and describe attitude of inquiry, with personal examples	Texts Articles Tutor Colleagues	Write a one-page synopsis of personal attitude of inquiry	Synopsis will be evaluated in terms of honest, open reflection of personal attitude indicating areas for improvement Due 1 April 2005

flexible so that changes can be negotiated as necessary (Crooks *et al.*, 2001). Your tutor or counsellor will guide you in developing and completing your learning plan. Table 1.2 shows an example of a learning plan.

Activity

- In your own words, identify and describe the key elements of a learning plan.
- Identify the essential criteria required for a sound, complete objective.
- Write one objective that you could achieve as the health-care professional working with Mary and Heather in the case study.
- Write a learning plan that you can use in your next clinical placement.

REFLECTIVE LEARNING JOURNALS

The literature contains many descriptions of reflective writing. Brown *et al.* (2001) distinguish between three terms that are often used interchangeably:

> *logs facilitate objective, scientific writing; diaries, written exclusively for oneself, engage the student in introspection; and journals represent diaries written for selected readers–teachers, mentors, peers, and/or colleagues (Heinrich, 1992), which include a reflective component (Landeen, Byrne, and Brown, 1992). Journals include both the objective documentation of logs and the personalized analysis and inquiry of the diary. (p. 141)*

A reflective learning journal is a written document that outlines your thinking about specific concepts and practices. A three-stage approach to reflection (awareness, critical analysis and new perspective) will help you write meaningful entries in your journal. When you are learning, it is helpful to consciously reflect on new ideas presented to you. Some students are encouraged to identify a concept of interest and to write about that concept in their journals. Often students begin by writing what they already know about the concept, what they have read about the concept, and perhaps outlining a number of questions that they may have. When you explore a new topic, you may not understand the terms or concepts used by the writer, so you need to seek answers from the literature or from an expert. Throughout your journal writing, you will be asking questions, explaining, disagreeing, trying to get to the heart of the matter, turning things over in your mind, and occasionally feeling a sense of frustration when you don't readily understand the concept. You can use your reflective learning journal to write about

- the process of learning;
- the insights you gained into a concept and how this new information has expanded your knowledge of a specific concept;

- the consequences of what you have learned;
- various clinical experiences and ideas about why certain responses occurred rather than other responses;
- the relationship between theory and practice relevant to specific experiences, such as why some theories work in practice whereas others do not;
- what you discover about yourself.

When learning about new concepts, your thinking may appear unclear or hazy at first. Don't be concerned. Expect a period of confusion when you are grappling with new ideas. Remember that learning requires time, energy and commitment. However, making notes in your journal can help to clarify concepts or practices and bring them into focus. Include your uncertainties in your writing and refer back to your notes to show that you are progressing in understanding concepts and how they might be applied in practice. The processes and interactions of thinking, writing, reading and reflecting will help to increase your knowledge of a specific concept or practice. Ultimately, this new perspective, gained with advanced knowledge about concepts, supports you in implementing appropriate skills in your own practice with older people.

Reflection sometimes requires you to stand back from what you have been doing and make a deliberate effort to think about it. Talking or writing can help. Here are some things to think about:

- What have you just done? Perhaps you have completed an activity on your own, read a chapter of a book, talked to somebody, or applied new learning to your practice for the first time.
- Why did you do a particular procedure the way you did?
- How did some idea or practice fit with what you have done before? Were you building on previous knowledge or learning?
- What was good and bad about your practice?
- How did you feel about the idea, situation or practice?
- What reflection made you think about your future practice?
- What were the consequences?
- How would you describe the situation?
- Why did a particular response happen the way it did?
- The particular response, how was it different from what you expected?
- What will you do next to continue your learning?

Reflection supports learning and ultimately your growth as a health-care professional. Be clear about the use of reflective learning journals:

- Will journals be written solely for student purposes?
- Will tutors read student journals?
- Will journals be marked?
- If marked, what percentage of the grade will be assigned to the journal?

- Will extracts of journal entries be shared with colleagues as a learning device?

Regardless of the answers to these questions, confidentiality of students' journal entries is paramount and should always be respected. Without confidentiality, there cannot be open and honest reflection, and the purpose of the journal is lost. Furthermore, there is a debate in the literature about grading reflective learning journals. Some writers caution against grading journals (e.g. Diekelmann, 2003; Holmes, 1997) and others support the grading of journals (e.g. Alm, 1996; Hodges, 1996). In keeping with these notes of caution, Mackintosh (1998) proposes that 'reflection is a fundamentally flawed strategy' (p. 553) and Cotton (2001) questions the 'hegemonic discourse of reflection in nursing' (p. 512).

Activity

- Describe how you will use your reflective learning journal to explore a concept of your choosing.
- Using the three-stage model of reflection described by Atkins and Murphy (1993) and applied by Scanlon and Chernomas (1997), provide an example of your learning on a concept from the case study of Mary.
- Identify three areas in which you are having difficulty with reflective learning. Plan to discuss these difficulties with your tutor.

PROFESSIONAL PORTFOLIO

Professional portfolios, or profiles, tend to include a synopsis of an individual's experiences and learning opportunities. The purpose of a portfolio is to provide evidence to support an individual's achievements throughout a career. Considerable attention is given to the development of professional portfolios in education and nursing (Borko *et al.*, 1997; Brown *et al.*, 2001). In both disciplines the portfolio provides substantive evidence to demonstrate competence in one's practice. A professional assumes responsibility for maintaining this documentation throughout a career, so it is important to establish an organized and comprehensive approach to collating significant achievements within one's professional practice.

Professional portfolios vary widely but often include a current CV, examples of learning plans and reflective learning journals, workshops or conferences attended, and perhaps papers presented, certifications, awards or special achievements. Moreover, a portfolio includes documentation of plans for continued professional growth. A health-care professional reviews this professional portfolio annually, replacing documents as necessary. For instance, a CV should be updated every year or, at least, when a change in position or other information occurs. Maintaining an up-to-date professional portfolio is necessary because many professional organizations require these documents to determine the competence of their members. In some instances the professional body may request the documentation be submitted for review and expect submission for audit within a 24-hour period. Retain a copy of anything you submit, just in case the material is misplaced or lost.

Activity

- Describe the main features of a professional portfolio.
- Explain how your professional portfolio will be organized to accommodate the essential components.
- Outline the planned learning needs that you will address in your professional portfolio to demonstrate your professional competence.

SUMMARY

Learning is an active and demanding process. Only when learners take responsibility for their own learning will they reap the rewards that learning provides to advance their competence and confidence as health-care professionals. Learning is enhanced through processes such as critical thinking, reading, discussing, and reflecting *in* and *on* practice. There is an obvious need for health-care professionals to engage in lifelong learning within the current health-care setting, fraught with numerous issues such as an ageing population. Future improvements in health care for all citizens will depend on professionals who realize the need for changing practices and who have the courage to change them.

Learning is the key to our future. Accordingly, Senge (1990) cogently expresses a perspective on learning:

> *Real learning gets to the heart of what it means to be human. Through learning we re-create ourselves. Through learning we become able to do something we never were able to do. Through learning we extend our capacity to create, to be part of the generative process of life. There is within each of us a deep hunger for this type of learning. (p. 14)*

◀ **Key points**

1 Problem-based learning is an approach to effective, meaningful learning.
2 Learning styles are diverse and adaptable.
3 Individuals tend to favour one learning style, but can stimulate the development of another learning style to expand their potential to learn from other stimuli.
4 Critical thinking encompasses five key elements: inference, recognition of assumptions, interpretation, deduction, and evaluation of arguments.

5 Critical thinking is essential for health-care professionals who are responsible for assessing patients and implementing care accordingly.

6 Reflective learning entails actively examining issues of concern in practice, giving meaning to those concerns from an individual perspective, and adopting a new conceptual perspective.

7 There are three stages of reflection: awareness, critical reflection and new perspective.

8 There are three levels of reflection: non-reflection, reflection and critical reflection.

9 A professional portfolio is a comprehensive document that demonstrates the current achievements of one's practice along with a plan for continued professional growth.

REFERENCES

Alm, C. T. (1996) Using student journals to improve academic quality of internships. *Journal of Education for Business*, **72**(2), 113–115.

Atkins, S. and Murphy, K. (1993) Reflection: a review of the literature. *Journal of Advanced Nursing*, **18**, 1188–1192.

Basford, L. (2003) Competence-based approaches. In: *Theory and Practice of Nursing: An Integrated Approach to Caring Practice* (ed. Basford, L. and Slevin, O.). Nelson Thornes, Cheltenham, Glos., pp. 470–482.

Borko, H., Michalec, P., Timmons, M. and Siddle, J. (1997) Student teaching portfolios: a tool for promoting reflective practice. *Journal of Teacher Education*, **48**(5), 345–357.

Boud, D. (1985) *Problem-Based Learning in Education for the Professions*. HERDSA, Sydney.

Boyd, E. M. and Fales, A. W. (1983) Reflective learning: key to learning from experience. *Journal of Humanistic Psychology*, **23**, 99–117.

Brown, B., Matthew-Maich, N. and Royle, J. (2001) Fostering reflection and reflective practice. In: *Transforming Nursing Education through Problem-Based Learning* (ed. Rideout, E.). Jones and Bartlett, Sudbury MA, pp. 119–164.

Cotton, A. H. (2001) Private thoughts in public spheres: issues in reflection and reflective practices in nursing. *Journal of Advanced Nursing*, **36**(4), 512–519.

Crooks, D., Lunyk-Child, O., Patterson, C. and LeGris, J. (2001) Facilitating self-directed learning. In: *Transforming Nursing Education through Problem-Based Learning* (ed. Rideout, E.). Jones and Bartlett, Sudbury MA, pp. 51–74.

Diekelmann, N. (2003) Thinking-in-action journals: from self-evaluation to multiperspectival thinking. *Journal of Nursing Education*, **42**(11), 482–488.

Duchscher, J. E. (2003) Critical thinking: perceptions of newly graduated female baccalaureate nurses. *Journal of Nursing Education*, **42**, 14–27.

Facione, N. C. and Facione, P. A. (1996) Assessment design issues for evaluating critical thinking in nursing. *Holistic Nursing Practice*, **10**, 41–53.

Heinrich, K. T. (1992) The intimate dialogue: journal writing by students. *Nurse Educator*, **17**, 17–21.

Hodges, H. F. (1996) Journal writing as a mode of thinking for RN-BSN students: a levelled approach to learning to listen to self and others. *Journal of Nursing Education*, **35**(3), 137–141.

Holmes, V. (1997) Grading journals in clinical practice: a delicate issue. *Journal of Nursing Education*, **36**(10), 489–492.

Hyrkäs, K., Tarkka, M.-T. and Paunonen-Ilmonen, M. (2001) Teacher candidates' reflective teaching and learning in a hospital setting – changing the pattern of practical training: a challenge to growing into teacherhood. *Journal of Advanced Nursing*, **33**(4), 503–511.

Ironside, P. M. (2003) New pedagogies for teaching thinking: the lived experiences of students and teachers enacting narrative pedagogy. *Journal of Nursing Education*, **42**(11), 509–516.

Jasper, M. A. (1999) Nurses' perception of the value of written reflection. *Nurse Education Today*, **19**(6), 452–463.

Kataoka-Yahiro, M. and Saylor, C. (1994) A critical thinking model for nursing judgment. *Journal of Nursing Education*, **33**, 351–356.

Kember, D., Jones, A., Loke, A., McKay, J., Sinclair, K., Tse, H., Webb, C., Wong, F., Wong, M. and Yeung, E. (1999) Determining the level of reflective thinking from students' written journals using a coding scheme based on the work of Mezirow. *International Journal of Lifelong Education*, **18**(1), 18–30.

Knowles, M. (1974) *Self-directed Learning: A Guide for Learners and Teachers*. Pearson Learning, Parsippany NJ.

Kolb, D. (1984) *Experiential Learning: Experience as a Source of Learning and Development*. Prentice Hall, Englewood Cliffs NJ.

Landeen, J., Byrne, C. and Brown, B. (1992) Journal keeping as an education strategy in teaching psychiatric nursing. *Journal of Advanced Nursing*, **17**, 347–355.

Liimatainen, L., Poskiparta, M., Karhila, P. and Sjögren, A. (2001) The development of reflective learning in the context of health counselling and health promotion during nurse education. *Journal of Advanced Nursing*, **34**(5), 648–658.

Loo, R. (1997) Using Kolb's learning style inventory (LSI-1985) in the classroom. In: *Proceedings of the Human Resource Management Division of the Association of Management and the International Association of Management*, **15**(1), 47–51.

Loo, R. and Thorpe, K. (1999) A psychometric investigation of scores on the Watson-Glaser critical thinking appraisal new Form S. *Educational and Psychological Measurement*, **59**(6), 995–1003.

Lyons, J. (1999) Reflective education for professional practice: discovering knowledge from experience. *Nurse Education Today*, **19**(1), 29–34.

Mackintosh, C. (1998) Reflection: a flawed strategy for the nursing profession. *Nurse Education Today*, **18**(7), 553–557.

Miller, M. A. and Malcolm, N. S. (1990) Critical thinking in the nursing curriculum. *Nursing and Health Care*, **11**, 67–73.

Myrick, F. and Yonge, O. (2004) Enhancing critical thinking in the preceptorship experience in nursing education. *Journal of Advanced Nursing*, **45**(4), 371–380.

National League for Nursing Accrediting Commission (2002) Accreditation Manual and Interpretative Guidelines Type. Retrieved 2 July 2004 from www.nln.org/testprods/ guideinterpretation.htm

Pierson, W. (1998) Reflection and nursing education. *Journal of Advanced Nursing*, **27**, 165–170.

Rakoczy, M. and Money, S. (1995) Learning styles of nursing students: a 3-year cohort longitudinal study. *Journal of Professional Nursing*, **11**(3), 170–174.

Rideout, E. and Carpio, B. (2001) The problem-based learning model of nursing education. In: *Transforming Nursing Education through Problem-Based Learning* (ed. Rideout, E.). Jones and Bartlett, Sudbury MA, pp. 21–49.

Rolfe, G. (2003) Reflective practice. In: *Theory and Practice of Nursing: An Integrated Approach to Caring Practice* (ed. Basford, L. and Slevin, O.) Nelson Thornes, Cheltenham, Glos., pp. 483–491.

Scanlon, J. M. and Chernomas, W. M. (1997) Developing the reflective teacher. *Journal of Advanced Nursing*, **25**, 1138–1143.

Schön, D. (1983) *The Reflective Practitioner: How Professionals Think in Action*. Basic Books, London.

Senge, P. M. (1990) *The Fifth Discipline: The Art and Practice of the Learning Organization.* Doubleday Currency, New York.

Staib, S. (2003) Teaching and measuring critical thinking. *Journal of Nursing Education*, **42**(11), 498–508.

Thompson, C. and Crutchlow, E. (1993) Learning style research: a critical review of the literature and implications for nursing education. *Journal of Professional Nursing*, **9**(1), 34–40.

UKCC (2001) *Requirements for Pre-registration Nursing Programmes.* United Kingdom Central Council, London.

Valiga, T. M. (2003) Teaching thinking: is it worth the effort? *Journal of Nursing Education*, **42**(11), 479–480.

Watson, G. B. and Glaser, E. M. (1980) *Watson–Glaser Critical Thinking Appraisal Manual.* Macmillan, New York.

Watson, G. B. and Glaser, E. M. (1994) *Watson–Glaser Critical Thinking Appraisal Form S Manual.* Harcourt Brace, San Antonio TX.

Wong, F. K. Y., Loke, A. Y., Wong, M., Tse, H., Kan, E. and Kember, L. (1997) An action research study into the development of nurses as reflective practitioners. *Journal of Nursing Education*, **36**, 476–481.

FURTHER READING

DeMarco, R., Hayward, L. and Lynch, M. (2002) Nursing students' experiences with and strategic approaches to case-base instruction: a replication and comparison study between two disciplines. *Journal of Nursing Education*, **41**(4), 165–174.

Lowe, P. B. and Kerr, C. M. (1998) Learning by reflection: the effect on educational outcomes. *Journal of Advanced Nursing*, **27**(5), 1030–1033.

Ruth-Sahd, L. A. (2003) Reflective practice: a critical analysis of data-based studies and implications for nursing education. *Journal of Nursing Education*, **42**(11), 488–497.

Scanlon, J. M., Care, W. D. and Udod, S. (2002) Unravelling the unknowns of reflection in classroom teaching. *Journal of Advanced Nursing*, **38**(2), 136–143.

Schmieding, N. J. (1999) Reflective inquiry framework for nurse administrators. *Journal of Advanced Nursing*, **30**(3), 631–639.

Smith, M. J. (2000) A reflective teaching-learning process to enhance personal knowing. *Nursing and Health Care Perspectives*, **21**(3), 130–138.

Thorpe, K. (1994) Decision making and problem solving. In: *Nursing Management in Canada* (ed. Hibberd, J. M. and Kyle, M. E.). W. B. Saunders, Toronto.

Ageing

2

OBJECTIVES

- Describe various theoretical perspectives on old age and ageism.
- Identify characteristics that suggest modern-day societies are focused on a youth culture.
- Identify sources of abuse to older people in family and organizational settings.
- Describe the concept of active ageing.
- Explain the role and responsibilities of health professionals in promoting active ageing.
- Identify policy frameworks that will support and promote active ageing.

POEM BY KATE

What do you see, nurses, what do you see?
Are you thinking when you are looking at me –
A crabbit old woman, not very wise,
Uncertain of habit, with faraway eyes,
Who dribbles her food and makes no reply,
When you say in a loud voice: 'I do wish you'd try';
Who seems not to notice the things that you do,
And is forever losing a stocking or shoe;
Who, unresisting or not, lets you do as you will,
With bathing and feeding, the long day fill.
Is that what you're thinking, is that what you see?
Then open your eyes, Nurse, you're not looking at me.
I'll tell you who I am as I sit here so still,
As I use at your bidding as I eat at your will,
I'm a small child of ten with a father and mother,
Brothers and sisters, who love one another.
A young girl of sixteen with wings on her feet,
Dreaming that soon now a lover she'll meet.
A bride soon at twenty my heart gives a leap,
Remembering the vows that I promised to keep.
At twenty-five now I have young of my own,
Who need me to build a secure, happy home.
A women of thirty my young now grow fast,
Bound to each other with ties that should last.
At forty my young sons have grown and are gone,

But my man's beside me to see I don't mourn.
At fifty once more babies play round my knee,
Again we know children, my loved one and me.
Dark days are upon me, my husband is dead,
I look at the future, I shudder with dread.
For my young are now rearing young of their own,
And I think of the years and the love I have known.
I'm an old woman now and nature is cruel,
'Tis her just to make old age look like a fool.
The body it crumbles, grace and vigour depart,
There is now a stone where I once had a heart.
But inside this old carcass a young girl still dwells,
And now and again my battered heart swells.
I remember the joys, I remember the pain,
And I'm loving and living life over again.
I think of the years all too few – gone too fast,
And accept the fact that nothing can last.
So open your eyes, nurses, open and see,
Not a crabbit old woman, look closer, see me.

INTRODUCTION

Kate's poem (Kate, 2000) poignantly reminds us of the stages in life as we unquestionably and unequivocally continue to age. The sadness, so eloquently depicted, is that old age is seen as something to dread, particularly when illness has removed one's ability to maintain independent living. Although Kate was suffering from dementia and near the end of her life, she was still able to write a poem that reflected her feelings and perceptions about how she was treated as a non-person. In Kate's opinion, the nurse was too busy and not really interested in knowing her as a person who had lived a rich life, gaining much wisdom along the way. Sad to say, these attitudes are commonplace in the health-care system, as evidenced in numerous reports of service failures. It is countered that there are many reasons for this position. Often negative attitudes are due to lack of knowledge and understanding of the ageing process and, in the absence of such knowledge, health-care workers continue to reflect societal values towards older people that often have negative connotations.

In his book *Learning to Grow Old*, Tournier (1972) was instrumental in awakening our collective conscience regarding the need to respect older people through the engagement of appropriate communication skills in order to acknowledge that they are valued and respected with the rights of being a person to the point of their death. To question whether older people have the right to 'personhood' beggars belief in the first place and is of concern to all of us given its potential reality. To begin to reflect on this position it is necessary to understand the notion of old age as determined by various criteria and contextualized within contemporary society.

Activity

- Take a moment to reflect on your own attitudes and values towards older people.
- Consider the media's portrayal of older people.
- Look at the caricatures that represent older people; consider whether they are negative or positive.
- If the media does represent older people in a positive light, is it because they are selling them goods or a particular lifestyle?

OLD AGE

The age criterion

Without a doubt, being old is a common feature of living in the postmodern world. Indeed, one of the greatest achievements of the twentieth century must be the 25 years added to life expectancy. Yet, future historians will reflect on this period and be struck by a society that was able to reduce the effects of biological ageing but that was ignorant or weak in addressing the nature of social ageing. Nonetheless, we have witnessed an aged society and, despite the doom-mongers, it is a moment in which to rejoice as these phenomena are set to continue well into the twenty-first century. The Organization for Economic Cooperation and Development asserts that in 2026 one in four people in the developed world will be aged 65 years or older (OECD, 1998).

The projections for the increase in the oldest old vary, but according to the 1996 US census, the numbers of people living beyond 80 years in 2040 will triple, reaching 26.2 million. In the UK, the 2001 census showed that 21% of the population was aged over 60, and by 2020 one-third of the population will be aged over 50. In addition, people over age 80 are expected to treble in the next 25 years and it is suggested that those reaching age 100 could be as many as 45 000 by 2030. On the one hand, there is reason to celebrate that advancements in health technology and improvements in public health over the twentieth century have focused on improving longevity; on the other hand, there is reason for concern that an increasing number of people reaching old age and advanced old age require increased support from governments to improve their quality of life and to sustain life. In the midst of these trends, we continue to grapple with a universal understanding of what it means to be old.

Chronological age

Being classed as 'old' is like entering an amorphous mass that is in itself multigenerational. Officially, having reached retirement age, most commonly 65 years, one enters the aged society. This classification continues to the point of death, which can be 100 years or more. Consequently, three, four or five generations cone under the umbrella of being old and, for official purposes, they are often treated the same. Grouping and labelling older people under one umbrella provides a time-oriented framework, but as Basford (2003) proclaims, it does not focus on the difference that exists between the young old and the oldest old in any meaningful way.

It is suggested that in becoming old one has reached the point in life where contribution to society's needs are minimal and that people of an advanced age are a burden on society (Basford, 2003). The truth of this understanding differs in that many early retirers are very healthy and lead active lives that often include public service, such as holding positions in local and national government as well as memberships of voluntary organizations. Nonetheless, there is evidence that the oldest old (octogenarians, nonagenarians and centenarians) increasingly suffer from health deficits that include reduced functional and cognitive capacity (Hoffman *et al.*, 1996). Notwithstanding these points, contemporary research recently identified that a reduction in functional and cognitive capacity is not an inevitable consequence of ageing (Butler and Gleason, 1985). Thus, procuring and facilitating healthy ageing is of paramount importance to all, given that an ageing society is already with us and is predicted to rise for the foreseeable future.

This phenomenon is indeed challenging government thinking on retirement age, social provision and pension support. If the age of retirement alters, as it did for women in the UK, then the classification of being old at age 65 will also change accordingly. From this position, age classification is a fluid and intangible notion. Nonetheless, there remains a point in a person's life, whether or not they are fit to continue to work, where the government classifies them as old. Having established this position, the situation is further exacerbated in that different terms are used to describe an old person that may have positive or negative connotations. Here are some examples: the elderly, old age, the aged, seniors, greying society, wrinklies, has-beens, and in the context of health care, geriatrics. In an attempt to avoid stereotyping and discrimination, the UK government has adopted the term 'older people'. Although not wholly satisfactory, it provides a universal framework through which older people can be homogeneously described.

BIOLOGICAL THEORIES OF OLD AGE

Chronological age is only one feature and its nature can be transient and crude. Therefore we need a description and an understanding of the physiological, psychological, social and spiritual nature of ageing as part of a separate reference framework, but viewed as an intricate part of the whole. The biological perspective identifies changes occurring at the cellular or subcellular level. Curtis (1965) holds the view that there are molecular changes within the body's cells as a result of spontaneous mutations, which over time become irreversible and accumulate with age. In simple terms, cells die through constant wear and tear, and this affects the functional activity of the organ.

Conversely, Walford (1965) proclaims that with age the body's immune system fails to recognize its own cells and attacks them as foreign entities (i.e. an autoimmune reaction). Over time this phenomenon affects people's functional and cognitive capacity. It is a picture that often typifies the caricature of older people. These theories can and do complement the chronological perspective of old age in that it is recognized that diminished biological function starts to come into effect after the sixth decade of life. The commonly held view is that with increased age there is a reduction in cognitive and functional ability. For example, there is a loss of memory, reduced skin elasticity, skeletal stiffness, diminished sensory functioning and reduced digestive ability. Such loss of functioning differs from person to person, but there is a perceived effect in the majority of old people that is directly attributed to cellular damage throughout one's life.

Activity

- In your learning journal, list bodily changes that occur through the process of ageing.
- Consider these bodily changes and, after wider reading and consultation with others, identify which of these changes are exclusive to older people.
- Identify from research findings how people can slow down the ageing process.
- When assessing people's age, what are the factors or characteristics that you look for?
- Having promoted health activities to the older person (losing weight, exercise and altered lifestyle), do you observe any notable differences? Do they look and feel younger? Why is this?

SOCIAL AND PSYCHOLOGICAL THEORIES OF OLD AGE

Other sources for identifying the phenomenon of ageing derive from the perspectives of social and psychological theories, which contend that no two people have the same psychological age, because they have different life chances, life choices and life experiences. The influences of our psyche and environment play a significant part on age and how we feel about age. This position is somewhat reflected in the adage that you're only as old as you feel. Chopra (1993) reminds us that an older woman recounting the tale of her first love can look and sound as though she were 18 years again, whereas a middle-aged man learning of his wife's death can wither into senescence in a matter of weeks. Cumming and Henry (1961) asserted that ageing was associated with disengagement.

This theory has been widely discussed and challenged by others, but it is a theory which attempts to explain that society and the individual interrelate with each other in a state of equilibrium. The process includes the notion that society and the individual gradually disengage from each other, resulting in mutual satisfaction and benefit. Thus, the older person prepares for death through disengagement from society by mutual consent. The individual disengages gracefully and with minimum disruption to the social order, passing on the power and authority to the younger generation. There is withdrawal from social roles, a reduction in social activity, and the severing of emotional ties with family and friends. However, the theory does not state whether it is the individual or society that initiates the disengagement process. Clinicians have noted that older people do in fact disengage from social intercourse and prepare themselves for death.

This theory has been severely criticized for encouraging negative aspects of social policy and attitudes towards older people. It did, however, provide a scientific template for the new twentieth-century practice of retirement from the labour force. This disengagement theory justified the rocking-chair lifestyle and the placement of housing schemes for older people on the periphery of towns and cities, supposedly to offer the peace and quiet of the countryside. Moreover, it could even be seen to excuse custodial forms of treatment in institutional care. It was a particularly dangerous theory because of its potential to become a self-fulfilling prophecy. If we expect and demand less of people because they are old, they are likely to conform to this expectation (Coleman, 1993).

Opponents of the disengagement theory, such as Havighurst (1963), suggested that the natural success of old age is to remain active, replacing work activities with new forms of activity that compensate for such losses. The argument here is that social disengagement is not the natural order in old age; it takes the view that disengagement is undesirable, promoting an unhealthy attitude towards old people. Social isolation and social inactivity should not be encouraged or supported, but social interrelationships should be facilitated to continue social integration that is complementary to the lifestyles and activities of the young. The key here is 'complementary'; for example, older people may have some physical dysfunction, but this does not detract from their ability to provide the wisdom that maturity brings to public service and policy making, religion and family life. In essence the level of activity changes to incorporate a more sedentary life but still affords internal worth and respect for what older people have to offer.

Although this picture reflects a sense of reality, it begs the question, why should the level of activity change? If older people are healthy, why should they disengage at all from work to which they bring a level of expertise? Why is it assumed that leisure activities are less active (e.g. playing bowls rather than football, watching dancing on the television rather than engaging in dancing themselves)? To some extent, this position can be explained by the socialization theory (Roscow, 1974). Roscow contends that in primitive societies the old accumulated power and authority through ownership of property, wisdom and levels of productivity. The young were, in truth, the dependants of such power but they provided physical support to the frail old in the position of social interchange with mutual reciprocity. In these societies, older people were revered and held in high esteem, thus they were given respect to the end of their days. Conversely, in modern western societies, the situation is largely reversed. Property, knowledge and new skills are held primarily by the young; the power and authority are therefore vested with the young and the old are viewed as a burden on society. Modern societies are youth-focused within strongly framed youth cultures. Roscow (1974) identified the following characteristics that lean towards the prominence of a youth culture:

- **Devaluation**: the status of the older person as a non-working, non-vital member of the social group, whose knowledge, values and general abilities are largely redundant, comes to the fore. This view is reflected in the wider social group's negative attitudes to older people, relative indifference towards them, or even overt rejection.
- **Stereotyping**: predominantly negative characteristics are often attributed to older people as a group. These opinions are usually strongly held and seldom questioned, even though they are largely unsubstantiated.
- **Exclusion**: older people are often actively excluded from equal opportunity for participation in many areas of social life (e.g. work, politics, community and recreational activities).
- **Role loss and role ambiguity**: previous roles such as worker, community leader and union official are removed but there is little activity prescribed or acknowledged for old age, except inactivity. This lack of a prescribed, required or recognized social role can generate as much ambiguity, anxiety and strain as the conflicting role pressures (e.g. between work and family commitments) of younger life. Indeed, younger people probably cannot even visualize what it would be like to have no recognized role in society whatsoever.
- **Youthful self-image**: in the absence of a clearly prescribed role and in the face of devaluation, exclusion and negative stereotyping, the older person sometimes rejects the older-person reality for a more tolerable self-image envisioning a younger person. This aspiration to youthful status indicates a discrepancy between the older person's perspective and those of younger people and even many other older people. This stance can lead to a strained relationship and older people being subjected to ridicule and rejection.

Following Roscow's (1974) characteristics, as described earlier, there are inherent pressures forced on older people to disengage from social activities even if this is not what they necessarily desire. Consequently, the process of disengagement from their former roles means that older people experience increasing social isolation and are increasingly devalued. No single definition prevails when discussing ageing or being old. Although there are some explanations given from a reductionistic perspective (i.e. chronological, physiological, social and psychological), each definition is a sum of the whole, in that people are individualistic, having a unique genetic make-up and life experiences that will influence their own ageing process.

Activity

- Identify the point in chronological ageing when individuals are characterized as being old and the reasons underpinning this phenomenon.
- Discuss with peers the physiological theories of ageing.
- Review psychological and social theories and recap how these theories relate to primitive societies and contemporary societies.
- Write in your journal how many older people you know who still engage with public life and/or are active in their communities. Compare them with individuals of similar age who have disengaged from societal activities.
- Consider how illness, particularly chronic illness, affects people's ageing processes and their ability to stay engaged with social activities.

AGEISM

Contained within policy and professional practice is the notion of 'ageism'. This perception occurred due to negative labelling and discriminatory practices that have become entrenched in society's views of older people. Slevin (2003) contends this position is due to stereotyping and prejudices that lack thought and/or foundation. Butler (1969), who was the first person to coin the term, emphasized that ageism was to do with negative action under the guise of discrimination within a particular social system. Discrimination takes several forms: victimization, physical and mental abuse, social segregation, and legal and moral sanctions. Slevin defines ageism as follows:

- It is directed towards a target minority group – older people.
- It is shared by the majority or is institutionalized.
- It is characterized by negative stereotypes – prejudices.
- It involves negative punitive action – discrimination.

Slevin suggests that defining a situation does not always prove that it exists. Arguably, there is a need to identify that there is a homogeneous group which has similar problems and that the group can be subjected to discrimination, prejudice and stereotyping. If older people come from a diverse group, those with power, authority and fiscal independence and those without them, then we cannot place all older people under the same umbrella. Victor (1999) asserts that, given the heterogeneous nature of older people, the term 'ageism' has only a limited value due to the lack of utility. Nonetheless, Victor claims that 'limited value' does not exclude its existence. Similarly, when applying the concept of discrimination to other groups (e.g. women or black people), discrimination does not apply to all but we do acknowledge its existence.

THE SOURCES AND ABUSE OF AGEISM

Ageism is a phenomenon of modern societies and has increasingly occurred as growth rates for numbers of older people have accelerated. Governments and professionals alike have originated the notion of ageism by expressing concern that older people will add to the burden on society's human and fiscal resources. Health professionals highlighted the fact that older people increasingly use the health system and block opportunities for others. Carstairs (1981) proclaimed that two-thirds of the oldest old would suffer disability and cognitive impairment and one-fifth would be bedridden. Embellished by the media, these statistics have helped to foster beliefs that all older people are, and will be, a burden to society. This has increased prejudice and discriminatory practices against the old, and society has generally forgotten to examine the reality and/or the positive contribution of older people.

The possibility that older people were being abused within the caring sectors came to public attention in the 1960s. Robb (1968) provided a plethora of examples of actual physical and mental abuse of older people by health-care providers in elder-care institutions. Examination of care quality and abusive behaviour within elder-care institutions continued throughout the following decades; it makes morbid reading and challenges professional practice within these environments. Sadly, four decades of evidence continues to highlight the fact that discriminatory and abusive practices are ongoing (Garner and Evans, 2000). Another form of discrimination is found in organizational decisions that deny people treatment based on their age. Thomas (1994) cites examples of many such incidents and challenged their ethical and moral basis. This age discrimination against needed health care is illogical and not based on scientific evidence. Currently, the position is less visible given the human outcry against it. Indeed, raising the public consciousness to such overt discrimination has been instrumental in government seeking ways to totally eradicate abusive practice. The government produced the *National Service Framework for Older People* (Department of Health, 2001) in concert with professional groups to readdress abusive and discriminatory practice towards older people.

Thankfully, institutional abuse has been identified and is being addressed. Unfortunately, as with child abuse, it is difficult to establish the enormity of abusive situations involving older people. However, we do know they exist as we have the term 'granny bashing', coined by the media to describe abuse against older people being cared for in their own homes by family, friends or neighbours. Having raised the public's consciousness on elder abuse (physical, mental and social), the media demanded action from government and professional agencies to prevent it altogether or at least reduce its occurrence.

There are many reasons why abusive behaviour occurs in the home; three examples are family relationships, social deprivation and financial hardship. However, from professional and organizational perspectives, it is suggested that prevention and minimization of elder abuse are hindered by lack of appropriate education and training for health-care professionals, lack of professional support systems, lack of respite care and lack of residential care. Identifying older people at risk has become an integral feature of contemporary practice and there is a growing body of evidence that such intervention models can be effective. Unfortunately, when elder abuse is occurring, particularly in the family unit, it is often masked by a conspiracy of silence. It is therefore the responsibility of all professionals to be alert for the signs of any abuse taking place. Having assessed that there is abusive activity of any kind, the health-care professional is obliged to take appropriate action to safeguard and protect the older person. Health-care professionals must always remember that, first and foremost, they are the patient's advocates.

It is clear that abusive and discriminatory practice will not disappear overnight, and it behoves governments, professional agencies and communities to develop appropriate policies to confine the problem or eradicate it altogether.

Activity

- Consider caring for an older person with challenging behaviour, 24 hours a day, 7 days a week without any respite. Consider how you would feel. Consider the help that you would require. Compile a list of known services that can help such caregivers and their families.
- Describe the needs of an older person who is in an abusive circumstance, remembering that it is often from their own sons, daughters or in-laws.
- Discuss the role of the health-care professional in preventing and minimizing elder abuse.

AGEISM AND NURSING

It is anathema to suggest that elements of the nursing profession are ageist, but unfortunately it is true. Several investigators have proclaimed that nurses do hold negative attitudes towards older people in keeping with societal values (Campbell, 1971; Slevin, 1991). Furthermore, through professional socialization the negative attitudes towards older people become more entrenched (Slevin, 1991), and for the most part, nurses wish to work more with children and young people (Campbell, 1971). The reasons for avoiding caring for older adults are manifold and include career aspirations and opportunities, the low prestige that the profession as a whole gives to nursing older people, as well as a lack of training and education that enables nurses to competently provide holistic care with people who have multiple health problems and who have a high incidence of complications.

It is not surprising that nurses do not readily seek to care for old people as a priority, given that historical patterns of care were founded on a dependent paternalistic model where the patient is a passive recipient of care. This model of care fostered old people to disengage with life itself and mark time until death arrived. These institutions became what Henry (1963) describes as 'tombs for the living'. The role of the nurse was as a caretaker of the body – washing, feeding, clothing, etc. – and is significantly identified in Kate's poem. Any meaningful communication was only minimally undertaken as experienced and reflected by Kate. The lack of holistic care and the promotion of active living can be seen as dehumanizing and at the heart of ageism. It is, however, laudable that a shift in approach towards caring for older people has occurred in recent times, and it is also true that most nurses provide care against a backdrop of kindness and empathy towards their patients. But we should be mindful that attitudes take a long time to change and not all care settings for older people are ideal. The lesson to be learned is that all people have the right to holistic care that is non-dehumanizing. It is only when this negative approach has been eradicated that ageism can be said not to exist in the nursing profession and the health-care system as well as in domestic settings and private agencies.

ACTIVE AGEING

According to the Brasilia Declaration on Healthy Ageing 1996 (in WHO, 2003), 'Healthy older persons remain a resource for their families, their communities and the economy'. Figure 2.1 shows an older person helping a small child learn through play.

The concept of active ageing has occurred out of the recognition that growing old does not mean you simply sit in a rocking chair and wait for death, but that you can engage in activities which will promote and

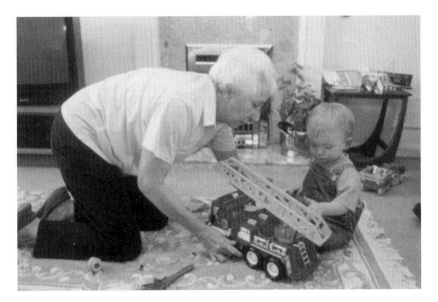

Figure 2.1

Generations at play

sustain healthy ageing, quality of life and life free from disabilities. Furthermore, it has expanded the thinking behind healthy ageing in that active ageing embraces the factors which include health care, human rights, independence, participation, dignity, care and self-fulfilment. The active ageing philosophy supports the disengagement from a dependent, passive model and recognizes equality of opportunity and rights of older adults in every element of life's journey as they grow older. It is recognized that, should they so desire, older people have rights to continue in political processes and community life and to be recognized for this activity.

This is not to say that older people currently disengage from community life, as evidenced in Spain, where older people, especially women, provide care for all age groups. Durán H, Fundación BBVA (in WHO, 2003) has calculated the minutes per day spent in providing care and illustrates how caring activities increase exponentially with age: '201 minutes if the caregiver is in the age group 65–74 and 318 minutes if aged 75–84 – compared to only 50 minutes if the caregiver in the age group 30–49' (p. 2). In Africa, in developing countries and in war-torn countries, older people are caring for children whose parents have died through famine, war and recently from the AIDS epidemic. The World Health Organization cites data that there are currently 14 million children under the age of 15 in African countries alone who are cared for by their grandparents (*ibid.*, p. 2). Although this makes morbid reading, it clearly illustrates how a significant number of older people continue to engage in an active life that is visible by its relative invisibility, but one that still contributes to the economic stability of society and socialization to life for a generation of young people.

Activity

- Write activities in your portfolio that you perceive as encouraging healthy ageing.
- Give examples of evidence from the literature that supports the notion of active ageing.
- Describe the ideal lifestyle and living conditions that would support the notion of active and healthy ageing.

What is active ageing?

According to *Active Ageing: A Policy Framework*, 'active ageing is the process of optimizing for health, participation and security in order to enhance quality of life as people age' (WHO, 2002, p. 12). The key phrase is 'health, participation and security' (WHO, 2002, p. 12). Through inference, it is suggested that older people have the right to engage in health participation activities so they can realize their optimum health potential that includes physical, psychological, social and spiritual well-being. Their continued engagement within society, life

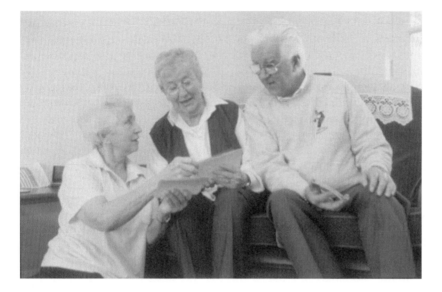

Figure 2.2

Sharing life experiences amongst supportive friends

and employment should be available in accordance with their 'needs, desires and capacities' (WHO, 2002, p. 12), and when health declines, older people have the right to expect that society will provide them with the basic necessities of life through care and compassion under the umbrella of security. The new paradigm is not to promote passive participation as fostered in recent history, but to generate the philosophy that it is accepted and encouraged to engage in active ageing activities that promote, maintain and restore health, and when health fails, there is a 'healthy' and dignified death. In essence this policy framework means enjoying an extended healthy life expectancy and quality of life that is free from disability. Figure 2.2 shows older adults enjoying quality of life.

In an active ageing framework, policies and programmes should embrace a holistic perspective that is interdependent and intergenerational and culturally sensitive. This approach facilitates the reciprocity required between and within generations so active ageing can be achieved and sustained. The ageing process as described in Kate's poem clearly illustrates how 'yesterday's child is today's adult and tomorrow's grandmother or grandfather' (WHO, 2002, p. 12). Evidence from social scientific studies suggests that the quality of life enjoyed in old age depends on life chances and life choices and the effect of the internalization process of those experiences. In addition, it relies on the way society adopts and encourages a caring philosophy as a central tenet in which succeeding generations provide social support for older people when the need arises.

A life-course approach

A life-course perspective of active ageing is an essential model if the deaths from early mortality and morbidity are to be significantly reduced. Moving on this notion, the Health for All policy frameworks for the WHO European region document (WHO, 1998a) identified key practices to promote and protect people's health throughout their lives and to reduce the incidence of the main diseases and injuries and alleviate the suffering they cause. Implicit within these statements are that all people are part of the health-promoting network; they are no longer passive recipients but active participants who are empowered to take responsibility for their own health. Non-communicable diseases (NCDs) are the leading causes of death in western societies. The major chronic conditions affecting older people worldwide are cardiovascular disease, hypertension, stroke, diabetes, cancer, chronic obstructive pulmonary disease, musculoskeletal conditions (arthritis and osteoporosis), mental health conditions (chiefly dementia and depression) and visual impairment (WHO, 1998a). These diseases are largely attributable to the modern world, given that previous prime causes of morbidity and mortality were associated with communicable diseases, maternal and perinatal conditions, and nutritional deficiencies.

Major attention to public health strategies was instrumental in reducing the incidence and prevalence of communicable diseases, maternal and child conditions, and nutritional deficiencies. However, the current incidence and prevalence of chronic diseases such as coronary heart disease, stroke and diabetes can be prevented if attention is given to individual lifestyles that may include tobacco consumption and other substance misuse, inadequate diet and lack of physical exercise. In addition, such risky behaviours are compounded through socio-economic status and living conditions (Basford et al., 2003). Given the increasing body of evidence that supports this kind of thinking, it is clear that attention to NCD risk factors is addressed from childhood to late life. Thus, policy makers, professional bodies and scientists all have a collective duty to design and implement policies and programmes that support active ageing.

Policies and programmes

Population ageing is a challenge to policy makers and others in the pursuit of maintaining health in old age. It is assumed that if policies significantly support active ageing there will be

- fewer premature deaths in the highly productive stages of life;
- fewer disabilities associated with chronic diseases in older age;
- more people enjoying a positive quality of life as they grow older;
- more people participating actively as they age in social, cultural, economic and political aspects of society; in paid and unpaid roles; and in domestic, family and community life;
- lower costs related to medical treatment and care services.

Such active ageing policies must empower individuals to take personal responsibility for their health while ensuring the environment is aged-friendly and that society values what is termed 'intergenerational solidarity' (WHO, 2002, p. 17). Personal responsibility means that people need to plan for old age and to make positive moves to engage in and maintain positive health practices. A healthy outcome is the main expectation; however, there is no denying that there are also fiscal benefits to society in that there are reduced impediments to continue work and there is greater potential for contribution to the workforce beyond the official retirement age. Longer, healthy working lives create a climate that would indeed offset the burden on society towards pensions and social support as well as those associated with health and social care costs.

Determinants of active ageing

'Active ageing depends on a variety of influences or "determinants" that surround individual, families and nations' (WHO, 1998b, p. 19). To achieve success, it is suggested that the determinants in the active ageing process must be fully understood before developing and implementing policies and programmes Notwithstanding, it is recognized that some evidence is yet to be scientifically determined, for example, determinants of role definition, role interaction between determinants, and relationship of pathways that explain how determinants affect health. Furthermore, it would be useful to understand how various determinants which enhance health have changed over the life course. Such insights would enable individuals to make healthy behavioural changes at points in their life that enhance quality of life and security in old age. We know that early infant bonding influences how we interact with others during our lives, we know how continuity of employment affects financial security in old age, and we know that access to high-quality health and social care is an added value in health outcomes. Finally, the

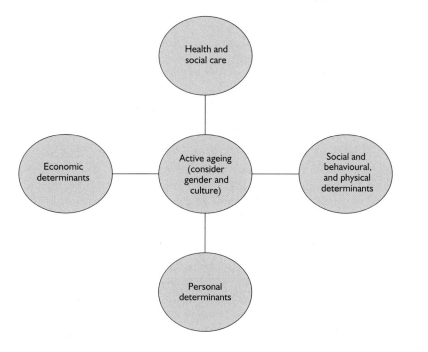

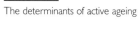

Figure 2.3

The determinants of active ageing

quality of our living environment has a significant effect on our health. We only have to consider the enormous damage to the health of the people who lived in and around the Chernobyl radiation disaster to understand how environment influences health. Figure 2.3 (page 35) shows the determinants of active ageing.

CULTURE AND GENDER

Culture

Older people are not homogeneous but very diverse. Culture is a significant factor when considering how people differ in their values, beliefs and spirituality. Indeed culture is pervasive and all-embracing, and according to WHO (2002), it 'shapes the way in which we age because it influences all of the other determinants of active ageing' (p. 20).

Cultural values, beliefs and traditions determine how we regard older people; for example, traditional cultures are more likely to accord older people due reverence and respect whereas, in modern times, western communities have lost this attitude towards older people. It is therefore an issue if co-residency with younger people is to be tolerated and encouraged. Cultural factors also impact on health behaviour, factors such as diet and attitudes towards smoking, gambling and drinking alcohol. For example, some countries have high tolerance levels for smoking within the privacy of their homes and in public spaces, whereas others are less tolerant. Notwithstanding, cultural attitudes and values do not always remain within a particular population or community. As countries become more multicultural, there is a fluid exchange of values and attitudes that permeate the mainstream cultural ideology associated with a particular country. In addition, there are universal laws that govern and sometimes override cultural values and attitudes, which include ethics and human rights.

Gender

'Gender is a "lens" through which to consider the appropriateness of various policy options and how they will affect the well-being of both men and women' (WHO, 2002, p. 20). The dominance over women in patriarchal countries continues in the twenty-first century and is evident in many of the war-torn countries around the world. In these settings, women have lower social status, fewer career opportunities, decreased access to health and nutrition, fewer political rights and lower education. Their roles follow traditional patterns as family caregivers and clearly affect women's health in old age. Some women are forced to give up their paid employment to undertake informal caring roles, hence their pensions are reduced to poverty levels. Conversely, men are exposed to other debilitating diseases, which impact on the active ageing process. For instance, men are more likely to suffer injuries due to violence, occupational hazards and risk-taking behaviour such as smoking, alcohol and substance misuse.

HOW ORGANIZATIONS INFLUENCE ACTIVE AGEING

In the twentieth century, the prime philosophy of health care focused on a reductionistic medical model framed around the concepts of 'cure and treat'. However, for active ageing to prevail, there needs to be a paradigm shift in thinking away from traditional models towards models that embrace health promotion and health education throughout the life course, disease prevention, primary care, and adequate provision of long-term and respite care. There should be no discriminatory practices and health professionals need to implement care with dignity and respect to all.

Health promotion empowers people to take responsibility for their own health, changing behaviour that is known, through scientific evidence, to reduce longevity and increase morbidity. Disease prevention is focused on preventive activities and management of conditions that arise more commonly as we age, particularly those diseases associated with NCDs and injuries. Preventive models include primary (avoidance of substance abuse), secondary (screening for early detection of disease) and tertiary (management of disease conditions).

The primary care model is a focus for most countries in the belief that it will provide the best solutions for older people and their caregivers with increased efficiency and effectiveness and with financial savings. Nonetheless, it is foolish to believe that acute care services will not be needed. The truth is that, for the foreseeable future, there will be an increased global demand for curative services and medication, but some of these services need not be outside the primary health-care sector, which supports easy access policies.

PERSONAL DETERMINANTS OF HEALTH

We cannot deny our personal biological and genetic make-up. As we write, the scientific world continues to identify genes that have the potential to influence the development of chronic disease. However, the environment also plays a significant part through the quality of housing, water, air, waste disposal, safe food and warmth. Thus, attention to public health is essential and cannot be overstated. The effect of social support throughout one's life is a compounding issue, and the lack of social support in old age can be quite catastrophic. In Japan, for instance, older people who did not experience social contact following the death of a spouse were 1.5 times more likely to die within the next three years than those with higher social support networks (Sugiswawa *et al.*, 1994).

Activity

James, who is now 100 years old, lost his wife 10 years ago; they had been happily married for 68 years. They had two sons and three daughters, all of whom died in their sixties. Out of 10 siblings, James is the sole survivor.

When he was younger, he had a strong network of friends, but they have all died. In his forced social isolation, how do you think he feels? Have you thought what it is like not to have the warm touch of another human being? Is there a strong incentive for living? Why has he survived longer than all his family and friends? Read what social scientists and gerontologists say about the phenomenon of living to old, old age without social support networks.

Key points ▶

1 There are several perspectives on ageing, including physical, psychological and social.
2 Kate's poem illustrates how a debilitating illness can often cause an older person to be neglected through various forms of abuse.
3 There is evidence of ageism and discriminatory practice towards older people within the family and in professional contexts. The reasons for this were elaborated.
4 Modern concepts and policies increasingly focus on supporting and maintaining active ageing so that the ageing process does not always mean dependent living; indeed many people live an independent life until the point of death.
5 Active ageing is now the subject of policy frameworks and directives.
6 Ageing is influenced by personal determinants of health.

REFERENCES

Basford, L. (2003) Gerontological nursing. In: *Theory and Practice of Nursing: An Integrated Approach to Patient Care*, 3rd edn (ed. Basford, L. and Slevin, O.). Nelson Thornes, Cheltenham, Glos., pp. 775–790.

Basford, L., Reed, A. and Nowatzki, N. (2003) Living Conditions, Lifestyle and Health: Cross National Study, EU Fifth Framework Project, Inco Copernicus Programme, Year 3 Report, *Diet in CIS*. Available from www.cordis.lu/inco2/home.html.

Butler, R. N. (1969) Age-ism: another form of bigotry. *Gerontologist*, 9, 243–246.

Butler, R. N. and Gleason, H. P. (eds) (1985) *Productive Ageing: Enhancing Vitality in Later Life*. Springer, New York.

Campbell, M. L. (1971) Study of attitudes of nursing personnel toward the geriatric patient. *Nursing Research*, 20, 147–151.

Carstairs, V. (1981) *Our Elders*. Oxford University Press, Oxford.

Chopra, D. (1993) *Ageless Body: Timeless Mind*. Rider, London.

Coleman, P. (1993) Psychological ageing. In: *Ageing in Society: An Introduction to Social Gerontology* (ed. Bond, J., Coleman, P. and Peace, S.). Sage, London.

Cumming, E. and Henry, W. E. (1961) *Growing Old*. Basic Books, New York.

Curtis, H. J. (1965) The somatic mutation theory of ageing. In: *Contributions to the Psychology of Ageing* (ed. Kasteorbaum, R.). Springer, New York.

Department of Health (2001) *National Service Framework for Older People*. The Stationery Office, London.

Garner, J. and Evans, S. (2000) *Institutional Abuse of Older Adults*. Royal College of Psychiatrists, London.

Havighurst, R. (1963) *Successful Ageing*. University of Chicago Press, Chicago IL.

Henry, J. (1963) *Culture Against Man.* Random House, New York.

Hoffman, C., Rice, D. and Sung, H. Y. (1996) Persons with chronic conditions: their prevalence and costs. *Journal of the American Medical Association,* **276**(18), 1473–1479.

Kate (2000) Kate's poem. In: *Professional Perspectives in the Care of the Older Person.* Emap Healthcare, London, pp. 176–177.

OECD (1998) *Maintaining Propriety in an Ageing Society.* Organization for Economic Cooperation and Development, Paris.

Robb, B. (1968) *Sans Everything.* Nelson, London.

Roscow, I. (1974) *Socialization to Old Age.* University of California Press, Berkeley CA.

Slevin, O. (1991) Ageist attitudes among young adults: implications for a caring profession. *Journal of Advanced Nursing,* **16**, 1197–1205.

Slevin, O. (2003) A nursing perspective on older people: the problem of ageism. In: *Theory and Practice of Nursing: An Integrated Approach to Patient Care,* 3rd edn (ed. Basford, L. and Slevin, O.). Nelson Thornes, Cheltenham, Glos., pp. 409–426.

Sugiswawa S., Liang, J. and Liu, X. (1994) Social networks, social support and mortality among older people in Japan. *Journal of Gerontology,* **49**, 3–13.

Thomas, D. (1994) Age related matter of care. *Elderly Care,* **6**(3), 5.

Tournier, P. (1972) *Learning to Grow Old.* London, SCM Press.

United States Bureau of the Census (1996) Population projections of the United States by age, sex, race and Hispanic origin: 1995 to 2050. Cultural Population Reports. United States Bureau of the Census, pp. 25–1130.

United Kingdom Government (2001) *United Kingdom Census.* The Stationery Office, London.

Victor, C. R. (1999) What is old age? In: *Nursing Older People,* 3rd edn (ed. Redfern, S. J. and Ross, F. M.). Churchill Livingstone, Edinburgh.

Walford, R. L. (1965) *Immunology and Ageing.* Springer, New York.

WHO (1998a) *Growing Older, Staying Well: Ageing and Physical Activity in Everyday Life.* Prepared by R. I. Heikkinen. World Health Organization, Geneva.

WHO (1998b) *Life in the 21st Century: A Vision for All.* World Health Organization, Geneva.

WHO (2002) *Active Ageing: A Policy Framework.* Retrieved from www.who.int/hpr/ageing/ActiveAgeingPolicyFrame.pdf.

WHO (2003) *Ageing and Life Course: News and Events.* World Health Organization, Geneva. Retrieved from www.who.int/hpr/ageing/international_day_en.htm.

3 CONTEXT OF MODERN PROFESSIONAL PRACTICE WITH OLDER PEOPLE

OBJECTIVES

- Describe the care of older people from a historical perspective that has influenced contemporary reforms.
- Describe models of care as a conceptual framework.
- Discuss standards of care relating to older people.
- Discuss political influences on caring for older people.
- Describe the influences of research and advancements in clinical practice.
- Discuss the need for education and training as preparation for professional practice.

INTRODUCTION

This chapter looks at the context of modern professional practice. The overall aim is to give you an understanding of caring practices with older people from a historical perspective that has evolved and shaped the care of older people in the modern era. Although many of these practices have outlived their usefulness, it has sometimes been very difficult to change professional and public attitudes towards older people. Nevertheless, over the past few years, some significant influences have enforced changes that place older people in a more positive and influential light. Chiefly they relate to the demographic success of the ageing population, social changes and the awakening of a social conscience towards older people, the promotion of active ageing policies, the empowerment of older people to take responsibility for their own health, education of health-care professionals in gerontological health-care practice, political persuasion and social policy relating to older people, findings from research and clinical practice, therapeutic and technical advancements, greater mobility of older people, higher care standards, and early discharge after hospitalized care.

In addition, the pressure for change has increased with each publicized service failure when caring for older people, through which current clinical and professional practice has been challenged. From a clinical perspective there has been a general sustained demand for changes to occur; this has encouraged a total re-examination of how care is delivered, and this has led to the creation of caring partnerships with patients and their carers, and within a multidisciplinary framework. In conjunction with these changes, professional practice has been charged with facilitating the empowerment of older people to take greater responsibility for their own health care: a model that departs significantly from the dependent (medical) model that has dominated health care within the context of the UK National Health Service over the past 50 years. However, in recent years there has been a growing emphasis to provide health care from a holistic perspective that considers the biopsychosocial and spiritual elements of human connectedness and interrelationships that significantly influence an individual's health and well-being.

This chapter aims to encourage understanding about the organizational constructs through which aspects of care are provided for older people, and it considers recent policies that have influenced professional and ethical practice.

HISTORICAL PERSPECTIVES

A review of contemporary health and social literature highlights the need for organizational and political reforms to address the needs of older people from a multicultural and multiracial perspective. Such a position is not an isolated or altruistic notion, but stems from years of social and political neglect and abuse of older people. (Chapter 2 describes the types of elder abuse and you may want to review them now.) Unfortunately, there is not a simple reason for this situation but a multiplicity of reasons that transcend all aspects of modern life. Here are some examples:

- It is generally expressed that when people age they increasingly become more physically, mentally and socially dysfunctional. This view is often portrayed through the characterization of older people in various media forms; consequently, it often becomes internalized as a position of truth.
- The prevalent societal attitude towards older people often considers older people as used commodities, a burden on society, and lacking in any usefulness in family or work situations.
- There is a generally held view that older people are apolitical, so their rights and needs are often neglected by political agendas. This position has been demonstrated by older people's relative invisibility in legal or policy documents.

To suggest these perceptions and attitudes towards older people have relevance only to the modern period would be unfounded. Indeed a review of history informs us that attitudes towards the older person have evolved and changed in accordance with social, political and cultural influences. Of particular notoriety in the UK was the landmark Elizabethan Poor Law Act of 1601, which raised the social consciousness of people and politicians towards the plight and needs of the poor, old and needy. The Act decreed that each parish was responsible for the health and social care of people residing in the parish. Of course, being old during this period was a relative position, given that the life expectancy was well below four-score years. The reasons for such an appalling situation were that women died from childbirth complications and people were often subjected to the effects of famine, pestilence and contagious diseases.

Life during these times was focused around day-to-day survival, and survival was threatened if people succumbed to illness or disability that prevented them from working and being self-sufficient. However, with the emergence of the Elizabethan Poor Law Act, there began to appear institutional organizations such as orphanages and workhouses to address the needs of the poor and needy. On one level, this law has an altruistic appeal in that it ensured shelter and work for those in need, but in reality the workhouses became notorious for subjecting inmates, particularly older people, to harsh treatment and work regimes. Once inside a workhouse, people rarely returned to where they had previously lived, except the local cemetery after their death. Death, for the inmates, particularly the old, was often seen as a welcome release from the drudgery and overwhelming worthlessness that existed within their daily lives. Sadly, the workhouses continued until the twentieth century, when social reforms and legislation brought about a new approach to address the health and social care of all people.

As part of the health debate, the UK saw the emergence of the National Health Service (NHS). The National Health Service Act 1947 offered a truly revolutionary framework through which health care was provided to all people, regardless of means and free at the point of need. Unfortunately, the speed of implementation of the new NHS denied the development of a truly ground-breaking organizational structure. Therefore the newly formed organization drew on the prevailing social and health-care systems that had evolved over long periods of time, bringing forth outmoded models of care, attitudes and therapeutic interventions that have supported and encouraged abusive and discriminatory practice, without the use of appropriate evidence. These approaches towards caring for older people often went unchallenged until they were drawn to the attention of politicians, the legal system and the media, ultimately bringing about changes.

Activity

- Go to the library or search the internet and seek out incidents of discriminatory practice, cruelty and abuse towards older people in institutionalized care settings.
- Examine the philosophy of care in your unit or trust, discuss this philosophy with your mentor and ascertain if there have been any changes in this philosophy over the past decade.
- Identify models of care that encourage dependence, then compare them with other models that encourage independence.

THE INFLUENCE OF AN AGEING SOCIETY

For several decades people have lobbied politicians to enact change through social and political reforms, but other factors have also brought about change. Here are the main categories.

The demographic success of an ageing population

The global phenomenon of an ageing society and the overall reduction of the young due to falling birth rates have provided a change in the balance of political power and persuasion. Politicians can no longer ignore the demands of older people and have recognized that, through the vote, older people can influence significant political and social change. In recognizing this phenomenon, it has been determined that older people are a source for social reconstruction and development. Ideas pertaining to this notion must include the guidance of policy development that serves to meet the successful adjustment to global ageing. In this context, the needs of individuals are considered as well as the economic contribution older people can make in the broader aspect of cultural and political life. The commonly held view that older people are a burden on society has at last been questioned in the knowledge that older people can, and do, contribute as proactive and valued members of society. The Audit Commission (1997) proclaimed that healthy ageing should be associated with adequate finances, preventive and active health care, and when health fails there should be the right kind of rehabilitative care and adequate support systems to ensure quality of life is maintained until the point of death. These principles require careful planning and sufficient human and fiscal resources that support high-quality and flexible health-care service. Figure 3.1 shows graphs of demographic and survival rates.

Figure 3.1   Graphs of demographic and survival rates

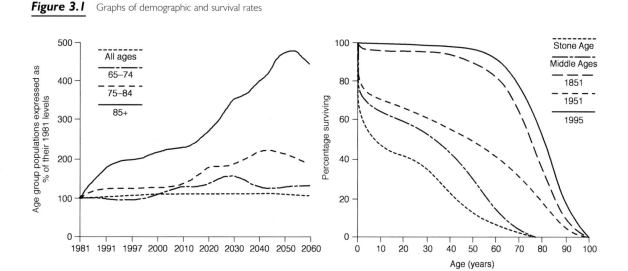

Social changes

Over the past 50 years social changes have made a significant impact on ageing and longevity. Attention to lifestyle and living conditions has had significant influence on individuals and communities. For example, lifestyle and living conditions include improved diets, smoking cessation, health and safety at work, increased interest in healthy living, and active ageing, and the reduction in communicable diseases due to better living conditions and inoculations. Older people are more exposed to the effects of social mobility, the impact of high divorce rates, single parenting, and the decline in the traditional family. These social changes have had an impact on the availability of social support from family members, and conversely, they have increased the demands on older people to continue with child rearing and child caring. Together this accounts for intra- and intergenerational support. Currently these trends continue to rise and the full impact of social changes has yet to be fully realized. For instance, we do not consider older people as sexually active human beings and at risk from HIV and AIDS, nor do we associate them with deviant abusive behaviours that include drinking alcohol and gambling out of loneliness, isolation and despair.

Health promotion and health education

The focus on health education and health promotion over recent years is an attempt to draw attention to people's lifestyles and living conditions that may have a negative impact on their health and longevity. Older people are now encouraged to pursue health-promoting lifestyles in the realization and knowledge that any degree of daily activity will enhance people's flexibility, prevent osteoporosis and improve people's mood, thereby preventing depression, and it will also offer more opportunities for social engagement, increasing social integration and creating opportunities for social support.

In 1999 the United Nations International Year of Older Persons (www.un.org/esa/socdev/iyop/) highlighted the link between poverty, deprivation and illness; it decreed that older people should be educated in correct nutrition and eating habits, that health professionals should be more aware of the health and social needs of older people, and that health professionals should extend their research to advance a greater understanding and knowledge of the effects of lifestyle and living conditions. This demand has driven the agenda for change in attitudes towards older people and the business of health promotion. Indeed Victor and Vetters (1988) clearly deconstructed the myth that it was too late for older people to alter their lifetime behaviours such as smoking, poor hygiene and dietary habits. Their research demonstrated that altered lifestyle can have significant health improvements even in their eighth decade of life.

Since the late 1990s, the focus of health promotion has been driven by organizations such as the Health Development Agency (HDA) and the World Health Organization (WHO). The HDA came into operation in March 2000 with a remit to improve standards in delivering health promotion and public health programmes. The WHO's mission is to reduce and/or eliminate the effect of poor nutrition, sanitation, housing, recreation, work conditions and environmental hygiene. In 1992 the UK Department of Health published *The Health of the Nation*, the first national strategy focused on health promotion (Department of Health, 1992). It was followed by *Our Healthier Nation* (Department of Health, 1999), which focused on five key areas that would prevent early mortality and morbidity from coronary heart disease, accidents, mental health, cancer and sexual health. Although these health-promoting activities focused on all age groups, there was specific attention on reducing inequalities in health that

- increase policies to promote the material well-being of older people;
- further develop health and social care services for older people to ensure accessibility;
- increase the income of the poorest pensioners;
- provide free eye tests;
- offer a national minimum standard of concessionary travel for older people;
- divide the costs of care between public funds and older people themselves;
- target adults to maintain independence through preventive strategies, partnership working between health and social care services, and support for carers;
- develop national standards for the care of older people.

Another noteworthy area is suicidal tendencies in older people. It is known that the rate of suicide increases with age. In comparison with young and middle-aged populations, older people tend to make fewer attempts per completed suicide, but use more violent methods. In addition, a greater proportion of males than females attempt suicide in the older population, and there is also a greater association between physical illness and suicide among older people. There are some known risk factors associated with completed suicide, and non-fatal suicide attempts; here are the main ones:

- psychiatric and physical illness
- being divorced or widowed
- living alone
- alcohol or substance abuse
- organic brain syndromes
- personality disorders.

Thankfully, health promotion and quality initiatives are now firmly ensconced within health structures such as the National Institute of Clinical Effectiveness and the Commission for Health Improvement.

Activity

Read about Mary's deep-vein thrombosis in the case study on page 205.

Empowerment of older people

Older people are empowered through education and the use of knowledge gained through the internet and other forms of technology. Individually, they are more knowledgeable about their rights as citizens and make appropriate demands; collectively, they provide a powerful voice through which their concerns can be heard by politicians at micro and macro levels. Contrary to popular belief, older people do not always vegetate in their retirement, but lead active and fulfilling lives. Furthermore, when illness occurs, empowered older people are more likely to embrace partnership models of care that give them respect and support for their independence and rights as human beings. Yet empowerment is not always easy to define; it is an abstract concept that lacks universal understanding and the concept has evolved through several disciplinary frameworks (e.g. philosophy, business management, psychology and sociology). Figure 3.2 shows a health-care professional encouraging an older person to participate in care.

Figure 3.2

Partnership in care

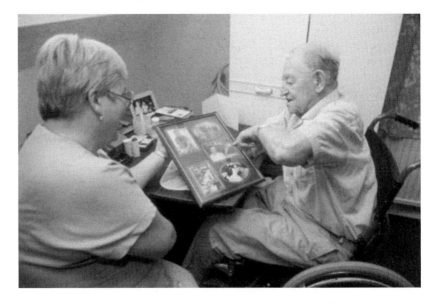

Development through this convoluted route provides a hybrid model that negates the opportunity for a simple explanation. Nonetheless, from a health paradigm, the empowerment model serves to transfer the power base from professionals to individuals or communities. The Patient's Charter was indeed intended to transfer power relations based on recognized collective need using the principles of enablement to advance an active response to oppression. Used in the context of psychoanalysis and counselling, empowerment serves to balance the power through the use of emancipatory approaches. In this context, the primary aim is to encourage a partnership approach towards care between the client and the professional, thus allowing the client to explore their social world. Holland (1992) offered a viewpoint on this form of counselling relationship based on the theories of social action therapy. Such an approach to counselling allows the inclusion of all aspects of the client's social world, with each representative being a stakeholder in the therapeutic alliance. Conversely, Rogers *et al.* (1997) examined empowerment as a conceptual framework for use with people having mental illness. Such thinking inspired the development and evolution of user groups, patient advocates and patient rights. Scientific thought on empowerment is currently polarized between empowerment as a process and empowerment as a product.

The product model is concerned with the promotion of self-worth, efficacy and an acquired sense of power (Dann, 2003). Wowra and McCarter (1999) extend this position, perceiving empowerment as gained and maintained through skill acquisition and information intelligence. On the other hand, the process model describes empowerment as a journey towards personal growth and enlightenment. Notwithstanding, Webb and Tossell (1994), cited in Jenkins (1997), perceive empowerment as a continuous process with neither an end nor a beginning. Within this context, 'being empowered' is measured through small steps that move towards empowerment practice. In this sense, older people, who are often disempowered through their vulnerability, can be acknowledged as empowered due to their own personal growth and development. In other words, this is a process of relativity (Kuokkanen and Leino-Kilpi, 2000). Conversely, Kar *et al.* (1999) contend that empowerment is a process through which health promotion can be achieved. For example, they claim that empowerment is the 'movement towards the powerless to take pro-active aspects of their lives' (*ibid.*, p. 1433).

Activity

- Read more widely on the subject of empowerment.
- Reflect on your own practice and ascertain activities that support empowerment as a process and as a product.
- Describe activities that support community empowerment.
- Identify activities that impinge on empowering practice or create a barrier towards empowering practice.

Enlightenment of clinicians in caring for older people

The education of health and social care professionals in the art and science of caring for older people in a sensitive, individualistic and holistic manner has added to the development of new holistic, individualistic and partnership models of care that support and maintain the notion of dignity and respect. Holistic care is concerned with a person's individual physical, psychological, social and spiritual make-up as opposed to the medical reductionistic model that perceives illness and its effect at the microcosmic level.

Micro and macro politics

The growth of a population of older people has significantly challenged policies that impact on health and social care, particularly policies that supported discrimination against older people and their pensions. Indeed a population growth of such magnitude presents governments with a real policy dilemma over the viability of pension schemes, public expenditure, implications for health and social care systems, and the risk of social exclusion for a large number of the population. Concerns like these are centred on the notion of a static economy and increased number of people seeking benefits from an overstretched social security system over a longer period of time (United Nations, 2003). Alternative models are being pursued with a refocusing on economic expansion and longer employment for those who choose it, in an atmosphere of support and collegiality. Attention to lifelong learning and transferability of skills is a feature of this paradigm.

However, while new ways of thinking are to be applauded, there are some areas that need attention, such as the effects of poverty, social deprivation and social isolation on ageing, longevity and quality of life. These fundamental issues are discriminatory to older people and deny them fundamental human rights. It is considered that attention to poverty indicators must be addressed if successful global ageing is to be achieved (International Association of Gerontology, 1997; International Year of Older Persons, 2003). The eradication of the poverty cycle for older people can only happen if they are fully integrated in the development and evolution of societies. In 2000 the United Nations Millennium Declaration (www.un.org/millenniumgoals) made poverty and human rights issues major components of the UN's goals and aspirations. It mandated that the number of people living in extreme poverty should be halved by 2015. Eradicating such poverty also means paying particular attention to the poverty that affects older people worldwide.

Dissemination of scientific research and evidence of best practice

Scientific research that supports older people in active ageing, restoration of health and maintenance of health has been instrumental in leading the way forward in attitudinal changes towards the older person and, indeed, with older people themselves. Three or four decades ago, upon reaching one's three-score years and ten, older people were considered to be (i) inactive, (ii) of reduced cognitive ability and (iii) unable to understand the world of politics. Today research has identified that many sexagenarians, septuagenarians, octogenarians and nonagenarians still lead an active life, for example, working, running marathons and competing physically with their peers

(United Nations, 2003). Others engage in sedentary activities that demand a level of cognitive ability or thought-provoking problem-solving techniques such as using a computer. Furthermore, new paradigms of care interventions have demonstrated that even when older people succumb to a major illness, such as stroke or heart attack, their health equilibrium can be maintained or improved with appropriate attention to active rehabilitation.

Therapeutic and technical advancements

We now live in an age of human part transplantation and human organ donation, something never previously encountered in human history. Technological advancements have made such interventions common-place, and not only is life extended by organ replacement, but its quality is significantly improved. In addition, there have been significant improvements in therapeutic interventions used in health care. In support of implementing therapeutic changes, there has been a growth in knowledge and understanding arising from investigations that have identified the evidence of best practice. Recently there has been increased attention on the development of genetic engineering that is poised to revolutionize health and health care in the quest to eradicate human suffering from modern diseases such as diabetes, asthma, some forms of cancer and hormonal dysfunction.

Mobility of older people

Older people are no longer immobile; they move to other countries and communities for pleasure, health, work and asylum and to avoid war, famine, drought and natural disasters. The social and health needs of these individuals are different, therefore health and social care professionals need to fully understand these needs from a multicultural, multi-racial and multifaith perspective.

MODELS OF CARE FOR OLDER PEOPLE

Historical caring models encouraged the provision of institutionalized care for older people. These environments promoted and supported discriminatory and abusive practice that denies individual privacy and dignity. Furthermore, caring practices were not underpinned by ethical or moral practice, or indeed scientific evidence. Over time these models of care have gradually changed, significantly improving the quality of care given within partnership frameworks and with greater understanding of the health needs of older people.

Contemporary practice has embraced the concepts of caring models that seek to illustrate theoretical constructs. Nursing, in particular, addressed this situation not only to assist in providing a framework of care but also to offer an understanding of nursing theory and practice. The following section briefly explains caring models and theories drawing on nursing paradigms as a way of explanation.

Activity————————————————————————————————

- Read texts that specifically address models and theories of care.
- Identify models that underpin activities of daily living.
- Identify models that relate to self-care and empowerment.
- Draw on your own experience and knowledge of caring models and reflect on their efficacy in practice.

MODELS OF CARE

In the process of making nursing into a profession, nurse theorists have often examined the relationship between theories and practice. In an attempt to understand this relationship, they determined and described frameworks or models through which caring practice can be directed and evaluated in a systematic approach.

Activity————————————————————————————————

- Read around the subject of nursing theory and nursing models.
- Examine the preferred model used in your area of practice.

Models can be construed as abstract thoughts as suggested by Fawcett (2000), who proclaims that knowledge is a linear process from the very abstract to the more concrete. Others, such as Chinn and Kramer (1999) and Meleis (1997), contend that the terms 'theory' and 'models' are overlapping, often interrelated with each other, so that distinction is difficult. Kaplan (1973) suggests that models are based on the expression of reality, such a model car or train. Focusing on the detail of the model is not without its uses, but there has been much confusion and misunderstanding over the past few decades. For many nurses, the plethora of information has caused them to reject the use of nursing models in the belief that they hinder nursing practice and the quality of care. Notwithstanding this position, evidence suggests that despite the confusion, it is generally agreed that models do afford clearer understanding of the reality of nursing practice. In *Theory and Practice of Nursing*, Slevin (2003) describes models that expand on the various concepts and explanations. Here are four examples:

- The physical or isomorphic model focuses its attention on the notion of reality; because of this perspective, it is often called the empirical model.
- The homomorphic model is similar to the physical model, but it differs in that its exact portrayal of reality is minimized.
- The symbolic model moves away from reality, often using numbers or shapes; it is often known as the theoretical model.
- The conceptual models are like symbolic models but instead of representing reality, they represent concepts or ideas.

It is generally agreed that nursing models are often conceptual models that provide a framework for understanding nursing practice. In explaining this phenomenon, Aggleton and Chalmers (2000) suggest that a nursing model is formulated around certain characteristics:

- The nature of people receiving (or about to receive) nursing care.
- The causes of problems likely to require nursing intervention.
- The nature of the assessment process.
- The nature of the planning and goal-setting process.
- The focus of nursing intervention during the implementation of the nursing care plan.
- The nature of the process of evaluating the quality and effects of the care given.

However, Fawcett (1993) suggests that a model

> *reflects the philosophical stance, cognitive orientation, research tradition, and practice modalities of a particular group of scholars within a discipline, rather than the beliefs, values, thoughts, research methods, and approaches to practice of all members of that discipline. (p. 13)*

The question raised is, how does this model differ from a theory? A theory, according to Chinn and Kramer (1999), is framed around a cognitive-empirical domain that explains aspects of phenomena, and the relationships between the dynamics of such phenomena. In essence, theory has a particular utility value that supports or prescribes our actions. As a result, theory can describe, explain, predict and may also prescribe.

Theory is concerned with phenomena that can be observed in a reality setting, and can be analysed in terms of how concepts are inter-related. In essence, theory is not represented in the abstract form as with models, but represents fully what occurs in the real world. Theory relates to the thought processes and scientific activity, thus fostering the process of theory construction in an attempt to make sense of the world in a continuous reflective cyclical framework. Merton's classic work *Social Theory and Social Structure* (Merton, 1968) identified these theoretical divisions:

- **Grand theory**: a general macro-level theory composed of abstract concepts in relationship, which is at the level of abstraction that facilitates description but is not capable of research verification.
- **Middle-range theory**: composed of less abstract conceptual frameworks, closely aligned to observable reality and thus capable of research verification.
- **Micro theory**: composed of empirical concepts that are observable in reality and capable of research verification. This type of theory can be a research proposition or hypothesis drawn from middle-range theory but usually not grand theory.

Although there is a clear distinction between middle-range theories and conceptual models based on various levels of abstraction, grand theories are very different. Indeed grand theories enjoy a similar reference framework to the frameworks for conceptual models. The distinction between the two is often weak. All this information may seem confusing, but it is refreshing to note that models and theories have provided a useful framework through which nursing and nursing practice can be described. Furthermore, they also enable the diversity of nursing to be understood and they explain how nursing can be developed. Indeed nursing practice has evolved from a task-oriented perspective to one that engages with the delivery of holistic care and one that encourages partnership working. The power relationship is often equalized between the professional and the patient, with the patient been empowered to take a shared responsibility for their health care. As nursing evolves and changes through the advanced scope of professional practice, theories relating to nursing and nursing practice will also change.

POLITICS OF CARE

With the increased focus on the care of older people, there has been a plethora of legislation that has centred on quality-of-life issues, and organizational reforms to improve the quality and standards of care that older people receive in all fields of practice. Here are some examples:

- NHS and Community Care Act 1990
- *The New NHS: Modern, Dependable* (Department of Health, 1997)
- *Modernising Social Services* (Department of Health, 1998)
- *Promoting Better Health* (Department of Health, 1987)
- *Working for Patients* (Department of Health, 1989a)
- *Caring for People* (Department of Health, 1989b)
- *Designed to Care: Renewing the National Health Service in Scotland* (Scottish Office, 1997)
- *Fit for the Future: A New Approach* (Department of Health and Social Services, 1999)
- *Saving Lives: Our Healthier Nation* (Department of Health, 1999)
- *Health and Wellbeing: Into the Next Millennium – Regional Strategy for Health and Social Wellbeing, 1992–2002* (Department of Health and Social Services, 1996)
- *Well into 2000: A Positive Agenda for Health and Well Being* (Department of Health and Social Services, 1997)
- *Towards a Healthier Scotland* (Scottish Office, 1999)
- *The National Standards for Older People* (Department of Health, 2001)
- Care Standards Act (Department of Health, 2000a) 2000.

All these documents focus on slightly different aspects, but there are some recurring themes and concepts. They address the health and well-being of older people and the standards of care that each individual person can expect in any organizational health and social care service. In essence there is a central political directive to improve the efficiency, effectiveness and economy that underpins caring activities associated with older people. Organizations are charged with operating a 'seamless' service that supports partnership working and better communication within and between professional groups. The following policies are mentioned because of their pivotal importance in influencing change.

NHS and Community Care Act 1990

The NHS and Community Care Act 1990 was introduced in two stages: (i) the NHS part was introduced in 1990 and (ii) the community care element was introduced in 1993. The central focus of this Act was to reform clinical practice. It encouraged caring for people in their own home environs and increased capacity for day care and respite care for carers. Assessment of care needs was properly managed with professionals who had the relevant knowledge and skill. The Act encouraged partnership working and the increase of private sector care, and it laid down the principles that assured the taxpayer got value for money. Inherent in the document were some key areas that are considered fundamental to the required changes:

- Multidisciplinary assessment with suitably experienced professionals.
- The involvement of local authorities as lead agents in the assessment process.
- The development of strategic plans for how care should be developed and delivered.
- The need for inter-agency approaches that support private care as much as possible.
- Older people in need are eligible for income support and housing benefit, except when in a nursing home or residential care and in receipt of DSS funding.
- Local authorities are charged with monitoring standards of care in residential homes.
- Social services are responsible for home help, respite care, day care, night-sitting service, and providing equipment to help people cope with day-to-day tasks.
- The NHS is responsible for district nursing services, chiropody, physiotherapy and supplies to assist people with incontinence.

The New NHS: Modern, Dependable

The New NHS: Modern, Dependable (Department of Health, 1997) is a landmark document that set out the government's agenda for change. This plan included the building of new hospitals and increased services in areas for the old, the young and for specialist areas such as cancer. There was a shift in authority and power from hospitals to primary care groups (PCGs) and primary care trusts (PCTs) in the belief that general practitioners and community practitioners were central to partnership working between secondary care and social care services. The PCGs and PCTs would address the health needs of the local population, promote health and well-being through a well-developed strategic plan, monitor performance and develop new ways of working that encouraged collaboration, cooperation and coordination of care services. In addition, the PCGs and PCTs have a duty to commission health services for their populations from the relevant NHS trusts and to be responsible and accountable for clinical governance.

Care Standards Act 2000a

The Care Standards Act 2000a identifies 38 standards that underpin the care of older people in care homes. The principal aim is to ensure that national care standards are satisfied to meet the needs, and secure the welfare and social inclusion of people who live there. The standards identified within the document are considered to be core, therefore the upholding and provision of these standards are essential requirements. The Care Standards Act (CSA) reforms the regulatory system for care services in England and Wales, and since its implementation it was deemed necessary to formulate a National Standards Commission to function as an independent non-governmental public body to address all aspects of health and social care regulation. Embodied in the title is the notion of 'standards'. These standards are clustered under the following umbrellas:

- choice of home
- health and personal care
- daily life and social activities
- complaints and protection
- environment
- staffing
- management and administration.

Each standard has an identified underpinning rationale and a statement of the intended outcome. The following broad themes are implicit frameworks that cut across all standards and have been especially sourced within the document (p. ix):

- **Focus on service users**: *Modernizing Social Services* (Department of Health, 1998) calls for standards that 'focus on the key areas that most affect the quality of life experienced by service users, as well as physical standards' (p. 48). The consultation process for developing the standards and recent research confirm the importance of this emphasis on results for service users. In applying the standards, regulators will look for evidence that the facilities, resources, policies, activities and services of the home lead to positive outcomes for, and the active participation of, service users.
- **Fitness for purpose**: the regulatory powers provided by the CSA are designed to ensure that care home managers, staff and premises are 'fit for their purpose'. In applying the standards, regulators will look

for evidence that a home, whether providing a long-term placement, short-term rehabilitation, nursing care or specialist service, is successful in achieving its stated aims and objectives.

- **Comprehensiveness**: life in a care home is made up of a range of services and facilities, which may be of greater or lesser importance to different service users. In applying the standards, regulators will consider how the total service package offered by the care home contributes to the overall personal and health needs and preferences of services users, and how the home works with other services or professionals to ensure the individual's inclusion in the community.
- **Meeting assessed needs**: in applying the standards, inspectors will look for evidence that care homes meet assessed needs of service users and that each individual's changing needs continue to be met. The assessment and service user plan carried out in the care home should be based on the care management individual care plan and, where relevant, determination of registered nursing input produced by local social services and NHS staff where they are purchasing the service. The needs of privately funded service users should be assessed by the care home before offering a place.
- **Quality services**: the government's modernizing agenda, including the new regulatory framework, aims to ensure greater assurance of quality services rather that having to live with second best. In applying the standards, regulators will seek evidence of a commitment to continuous improvement, quality services, support, accommodation, and facilities that ensure a good quality of life and health for service users.
- **Quality workforce**: competent, well-trained managers and staff are fundamental to achieving good quality care for service users. Topss (Training Organization for the Personal and Social Services), is developing national occupational standards for care staff, including induction competences and foundation programmes. In applying the standards, regulators will look for evidence that registered managers and staff achieve Topss requirements, and comply with any code of practice published by the General Social Care Council.

National Service Framework for Older People

The *National Service Framework for Older People* (NSFOP) is part of a series of standard-setting frameworks that target chronic diseases, mental health, cancer, and the health and well-being of children (Department of Health, 2003). The list continues to grow and ultimately it will reflect all major areas of health care that impact on early mortality and morbidity. The national frameworks have evolved out of the need to improve the efficiency, effectiveness and economic service that meets the needs of all clients and patients. These inherent features are identified in the government's *National Health Service Ten-Year Plan* (Department of Health, 2000b). The plan is framed around some key principles that ensure the NHS will provide

- a universal service based on clinical need, not ability to pay;
- a comprehensive service to meet the complex needs of older people;
- individualized and culturally sensitive services for people and their carers;
- standards of service that will be audited and monitored;
- a model for integrating health and social care services that will become 'seamless';
- infrastructures that promote health and enhance the quality of life for older people.

The standards identified in the NSFOP have reflected these sentiments and have built on previous legislation and policy documents, such as the CSA. The document is itself very comprehensive but here are some examples of the priorities it identifies.

Rooting out discrimination
Rooting out age discrimination has commenced with changing attitudes and policies within the very essence of NHS organizations. Each organization is required to ensure there is a fair access to services that is purely based on clinical evidence. Evidence that age-discriminatory practice is changing can be illustrated by the fact that 'between 2000 and 2002 breast cancer surgery for patients 85 and over rose by 13%. Coronary artery bypass grafts increased by 16% for those aged 65 or over, and an increase of 32% among patients aged 75 or over and 65% in the 85 plus age group' (Department of Health, 2003, p. 11). Furthermore, some hospitals have appointed nurses as champions to root out age discrimination in the ward areas; others are applying stringent audit practices that involve older people in the identification of age discrimination.

Person-centred care
Person-centred care draws on the desires, needs and wants of older people. NHS audits are concerned with measuring user involvement to express their experience of the caring journey that includes 'access, respect and dignity, information and education, involvement and choice, physical and emotional needs, coordination of care, environment and facilities, health improvement and community involvement' (Department of Health, 2003, p. 15). In addition, there is an active promotion of an integrative health-care provision that encourages a single assessment, joint coordinated care responsibility, and one that works towards improving the quality of care.

Intermediate care
Intermediate care provides a new dimension of care service that will enable older people to have intermediate care within their own home environment, or designated care setting, with the principal aim of promoting independent living.

Stroke

Preventing strokes will be a priority for the NHS, but when a stroke has occurred, specialist stroke services will be available. The primary aim is to improve the health outcome of patients who have suffered from stroke through the use of specialist stroke teams in dedicated care settings. In Sheffield the stroke service now has 84 dedicated beds as well as a comprehensive community-based rehabilitation service that provides an alternative to hospital-based treatment. In Newcastle, stroke patients can choose rehabilitation at home or in the gym, with support from specialist physiotherapists.

Falls

The NHS, working in partnership with councils, will seek to prevent falls and resultant fractures in the older population. When the older person has succumbed to a fall, effective treatment will be given, followed by rehabilitation services if required. Falls are the major cause of disability and the leading cause of mortality in people aged 75 years and over. Many organizations have arranged expert multidisciplinary 'falls' teams to reduce the number of incidences and improve patient outcomes. Examples of good practice are identification and treatment of older people with osteoporosis, active falls prevention services and proactive use of risk assessment.

Mental health in older people

Mental health services will be maximized to provide a comprehensive, integrated service for older people suffering from mental ill health. Preventing, treating and managing mental illness in older people are primary concerns given that there is an increased number of older people with dementia and depression. For example, about 5% of the population over 65 has dementia and 10–15% over 65 will be clinically depressed (Department of Health, 2003, p. 33).

Promoting an active, healthy life

Health promotion will be offered at all stages of the age span to encourage a healthy, active, independent life, thus reducing the need for support from families and health and social care services (Department of Health, 2000a, p. 14). Examples of good practice include Rotherham's IT2Eat, which aims to provide older people with advice on diet and healthy eating. It does this not only through nutrition classes but also by teaching older people the principles of internet shopping. Healthy eating advice is also available on the project's own website. Participants receive second-hand computers and modems, which are then installed in their own homes to enable their participation with the programme. The oldest user is 98 years old (Department of Health, 2003).

Improving medicines management for older people

The standard stipulates that people over the age of 75 should normally have their medicines reviewed at least annually and those taking four or more medicines should have a review every six months.

Multidisciplinary care

Multidisciplinary care is considered to be a model that ensures the needs of older people are met. Champions in the form of specialist nurse, or the modern matron, have been identified to encourage multi-disciplinary working practices that benefit older people. Furthermore, it is decreed that working partnerships between health and social care organizations must be developed in the spirit of cooperation and the promotion of independent living for older people. For example, between 2000/01 and 2001/02 intensive home care increased by 5100 from 72 300 to 77 400 (Department of Health, 2003, p. 23) and primary care services have been improved to meet the expectations and demands of older people.

Competent workforce

Older people should have their health care delivered by a competent workforce that has the knowledge, skill, understanding and experience to deliver high-quality care.

MONITORING AND ASSURING QUALITY OF CARE

The policy documents cited earlier demand changes in service provision and delivery. In addition, these policy documents have called for greater professional accountability and quality assurance. The Commission for Health Improvement and the emphasis on clinical governance seek to address quality and accountability from a legal perspective.

The Commission for Health Improvement

The Health Act 1999 and its associated regulations identified the need to establish the Commission for Health Improvement (CHI), through which health-care agencies and organizations are accountable for their actions. The drive for these developments came from the numerous reports of service failure, the lack of professional competence, and archaic models of practice that were not backed by sound evidence. The CHI came into operation on 1 April 2000 with a clear mandate to ensure every patient and client receives the same standard of care from competent professionals. It seeks to assure, monitor and improve the quality of care by undertaking clinical governance reviews. In addition, the CHI is required to investigate service failure through a rapid response and base its findings on sound evidence. The CHI operates on six principles:

- The patient's experience is at the heart of CHI's work.
- CHI will be independent, rigorous and fair.
- CHI's approach is developmental and will support the NHS to continuously improve.
- CHI's work will be based on the best available evidence and focus on improvement.
- CHI will be open and accessible.

- CHI will apply the same standards of continuous improvement to itself that it expects of others.

Clinical governance

Central to the work of the CHI is the need to examine every aspect of clinical governance to improve the quality of care for patients and clients. Clinical governance is a framework through which health agencies and organizations are accountable for their actions and the standards of care they provide. The Department of Health (2001, p. 1) has described systems and processes for the monitoring and improvement of services:

- consultation and patient involvement
- clinical risk management
- clinical audit
- research and effectiveness
- staffing and staff management
- education, training and continual personal and professional development
- the use of information about patients' experiences, outcomes and processes.

Clinical governance aims to improve the quality of life, and health, of the patient. In part, it provides mechanisms to protect patients and NHS professionals by making sure hospitals and community organizations develop structures to improve the quality of care. It aims to instil confidence by ensuring a safe clinical environment in which to 'accommodate rising patient dependency, and shorter hospital stays attributed to the ageing population' (Department of Health, 1997, p. xx). Implementing the processes of clinical governance shifts the emphasis away from reactive care and towards proactive care, such as prevention. Furthermore, clinical governance seeks to ensure that clinical practice is patient-centred and underpinned by sound evidence; that there is a continuous improvement of patient services and care; and that there is a transparent openness through which mistakes are addressed and rectified as well as a commitment to learning from these mistakes.

Practice and professional development

Clinical governance is about ensuring that health-care professionals have the correct knowledge, skills and competence to undertake a particular role efficiently and effectively. This means that health-care professionals have a duty to continue learning throughout their career so they are always competent to practise. Lifelong learning is an individual task, but team competence also needs to be addressed, and other workers' learning needs to be considered in the spirit of caring partnerships.

Education and training

The need for an educated and competent workforce has been identified in many policy documents on the care of older people. Knowledge acquisition does not stop after entering the profession, but continues throughout your career. This principle is embedded in the legal requirement to demonstrate competence in your field of practice at each point of re-registration (every three years in nursing); it is the principle of lifelong learning. The Department of Health contends that:

> *Lifelong learning is about growth and opportunity about making sure that our staff, the teams and organizations they relate to, and work in, can acquire new knowledge and skills, both to realize their potential and help shape and change things for the better. (Department of Health, 2001, p. 1)*

Central to the notion of lifelong learning is the recognition that patients and their families will benefit from a workforce that is suitably qualified and fit to practise in a dynamic health-care system. To support learning, organizations are now adopting support systems and resources and they facilitate learning opportunities that are patient-centred and clinically based, with the appropriate evidence identified. Furthermore, they encourage learning through personal reflection and a team structure. Educational opportunities will be formal and informal but they will try to advance professional understanding of the older person's health and social care needs. Curricula should determine the range and depth of knowledge and skill acquisition required for the care of older people. They should reflect diversity issues; ethical and legal issues; the biopsychosocial and spiritual aspects of care; pharmacology; therapeutic interventions, including orthodox and complementary therapies; social policy; and the sociological and psychological aspects of the ageing phenomenon.

SUMMARY

Professional practice is always contextualized within the frameworks of contemporary society. As societies evolve and change, so do the developments of professional practice and organizational structures. Nonetheless, evolutionary progress engages new concepts while drawing from concepts that are embedded in historical perspectives. Health care follows this form of lineage and sometimes forgets to let go of outdated and outmoded forms of practice, something which harms patients rather than doing good. For the most part, changes in practice can be seen as insipid and almost invisible, but sometimes they can be radical in nature, as within revolutions or major social reforms. Change is directed through technological developments, research findings, therapeutic developments, social pressure, epidemiology, demography and changes in caring practices.

Changes in caring practice for older people have occurred due to the success of an ageing population; political directives that have arisen from public scrutiny of numerous service failures; abusive and archaic caring practices; active ageing programmes; empowerment, knowledge advancement of health-care professionals and greater skill acquisition. Each professional group has advanced its knowledge and understanding of older people and their health-care needs using models and theories that explain the nature of people receiving care, health-care problems and associated aetiology, assessment, planning, intervention and the process of evaluating the quality and health outcomes.

The modern approaches towards care are directly influenced by legislation and policy. Over recent years a plethora of documents have considered social, political and health-care reform. This chapter has highlighted some of the major policies and the guidance they give on standards of care, professional practice, targets to reduce diseases, and illnesses identified as major contributors to early mortality and morbidity. Within all forms of standard-setting there is a need to organize and implement a sophisticated framework through which standards can be monitored and evaluated so that quality of care can be assured. In this context, the Commission for Health Improvement is acknowledged for its role in monitoring standards and for examining every aspect of clinical governance through which quality of care is enhanced. Such models of practice may appear overly bureaucratic, but evidence suggests that there have been significant improvements in care towards older people and that standards of care continue to rise.

◀ **Key points**

1 Former abusive and negative attitudes towards older people have been addressed through policy and changes in social attitude.
2 An increase in the ageing population, advancing technology, scientific discoveries and the need to improve quality of life have stimulated political action.
3 The focus on the ageing population has led to improved standards in all aspects of health and social care.
4 Research activity continues to provide evidence for challenging current practices.
5 The complexity of caring for older people requires well-educated and competent health-care professionals who provide safe, ethical and competent care.
6 The continually changing health-care arena demands each professional to take responsibility for lifelong learning.

REFERENCES

Aggleton, P. and Chalmers, H. (2000) *Nursing Models and Nursing Practice*, 2nd edn. Macmillan, Basingstoke.

Audit Commission (1997) *The coming of age: improving care services for older people*. Audit Commission, London.

Chinn, P. L. and Kramer, M. K. (1999) *Theory and Nursing: A Systematic Approach*. Mosby, St Louis IL.

Dann, K. (2003) Empowering care. In: *Theory and Practice of Nursing: An Integrated Approach to Patient Care*, 2nd edn (ed. Basford, L. and Slevin, O.). Nelson Thornes, Cheltenham, Glos., pp. 63–83.

Department of Health (1947) *The National Health Service Act*. The Stationery Office, London.

Department of Health (1987) *Promoting Better Health*. The Stationery Office, London.

Department of Health (1989a) *Working for Patients*. The Stationery Office, London.

Department of Health (1989b) *Caring for People*. The Stationery Office, London.

Department of Health (1990) *The NHS and Community Care Act*. The Stationery Office, London.

Department of Health (1992) *The Health of the Nation*. The Stationery Office, London.

Department of Health (1997) *The New NHS: Modern, Dependable*. The Stationery Office, London.

Department of Health (1998) *Modernising Social Services*. The Stationery Office, London.

Department of Health (1999) *Saving Lives: Our Healthier Nation*. The Stationery Office, London.

Department of Health (2000a) *Care Standards Act*. The Stationery Office, London.

Department of Health (2000b) *National Health Service Ten-Year Plan*. The Stationery Office, London.

Department of Health (2001) *National Service Framework for Older People*. The Stationery Office, London.

Department of Health and Social Services (1996) *Health and Wellbeing: Into the Next Millennium – Regional Strategy for Health and Social Wellbeing (1992–2002)*. DHSS, Belfast.

Department of Health and Social Services (1997) *Well into 2000: A Positive Agenda for Health and Wellbeing*. DHSS, Belfast.

Department of Health and Social Services (1999) *Fit for the Future – A New Approach*. DHSS, Belfast.

Fawcett, J. (1993) *Analysis and Evaluation of Nursing Theories*. F. A. Davis, Philadelphia IL.

Fawcett, J. (2000) *Analysis and Evaluation of Contemporary Nursing Knowledge: Nursing Models and Theories*. F. A. Davis, Philadelphia PA.

Holland, S. (1992) From social abuse to social action: a neighbourhood psychotherapy and social action project for women. In: *Gender Issues in Clinical Psychology* (ed. Ussher, J. M. and Nicolson, P.). Routledge, London.

International Association of Gerontology (1997) Adelaide declaration on ageing. Retrieved on 22 April 2004 from www.sfu.ca/iag/publications/adelaide.htm.

Jenkins, R. (1997) Issues of empowerment for nurses and clients. *Nursing Standard*, 11(46), 44–46.

Kaplan, A. (1973) *The Conduct of Inquiry*. Intertext Books, Aylesbury.

Kar, S. B., Pascual, C. and Chickering, K. (1999) Empowerment of women for health promotion: a meta-analysis. *Social Science and Medicine*, 49(11), 1431–1460.

Kuokkanen, L. and Leino-Kilpi, H. (2000) Power and empowerment in nursing: three theoretical approaches. *Journal of Advanced Nursing*, 31(1), 235–241.

Meleis, A. I. (1997) *Theoretical Nursing: Development and Progress*, 3rd edn. Lippincott, New York.

Merton, R. K. (1968) *Social Theory and Social Structure*. Free Press, New York.

Rogers, S., Chamberlin, J., Langer Ellison, M. *et al.* (1997) A consumer-constructed scale to measure empowerment among users of mental health services. *Psychiatric Services*, 48(8), 1042–1047.

Scottish Office (1997) *Designed to Care: Renewing the National Health Service in Scotland*. The Stationery Office, Edinburgh.

Scottish Office (1999) *Towards a Healthier Scotland*. The Stationery Office, Edinburgh.

Slevin, O. (2003) Nursing models and theories: major contributions. In: *Theory and Practice of Nursing: An Integrated Approach to Patient Care*, 2nd edn (ed. Basford, L. and Slevin, O.). Nelson Thornes, Cheltenham, Glos., pp. 255–283.

United Nations (2003) *International Year of Older Persons*. United Nations, Geneva.

Victor, C. R. and Vetters, N. J. (1988) Preparing the elderly for discharge from hospital: a neglected aspect of care. *Age and Ageing*, 17(3), 155–163.

Webb, R. and Tossell, D. (1994) *Inside the Caring Services*, 2nd edn. Edward Arnold, London. Cited in: Jenkins, R. (1997) Issues of empowerment for nurses and clients. *Nursing Standard*, 11 (46), 44–46.

Wowra, S. and McCarter, R. (1999) Validation of the empowerment scale with an outpatient mental health population. *Psychiatric Services*, 50(7), 959–996.

4 YOU AS A PROFESSIONAL PRACTITIONER WITH OLDER PEOPLE

OBJECTIVES

- Discuss the requirements for becoming a registered nurse.
- Review and explain professional responsibility and accountability.
- Describe the major tenets of the Code of Professional Conduct and compare this code to codes affecting others who provide services to older patients.
- Describe specific skills that nurses need for working with older people.
- Discuss issues related to providing care for older people, including how to resolve ethical and legal issues involving care and treatment for older people.

INTRODUCTION

Professional practice demands a legal duty, responsibility and accountability. Dictionaries describe a profession that is underpinned by advanced knowledge that requires long and intensive academic preparation. This description falls short of modern interpretations whereby a profession is framed around certain characteristics that draw on a specific body of knowledge that is supported by evidence from scientific research or practice. Each profession is governed by statutory legislation and core competencies for practice are predetermined. Here 'competence' refers to the relevant knowledge, skill, understanding, experience and ethical considerations.

Furthermore, in the context of health care, there is a requirement that there is an altruistic attitude towards community service, thus minimizing the risk of the abuse of professional power or privileged information (Basford, 2003). Vollmer and Mills (1966) suggest that there is an evolutionary nature of occupational groups as they strive to become a profession, moving along a continuous abstract line from non-professional to professional status as they embrace each characteristic that identifies professional practice. Having reached a point on this line where it is assumed that certain professional characteristics have been achieved, then rights and obligations are conferred on the occupational group, commensurate with professional recognition. Chiefly these rights relate to autonomy, responsibility, accountability, monopoly and rewards:

- Autonomy assumes that society acknowledges the professional group has a specialist body of knowledge and skill.
- They have the right to govern their own activities and produce and review their professional standards and codes of conduct.

- Accountability means that they are responsible and accountable for their own actions.
- Responsibility means they have a professional responsibility to act in the interest of individuals and society, doing no harm, and where necessary acting as advocates.
- Monopoly refers to the fact that the professional group has a specific body of knowledge and skill that is unique. They are afforded protection through laws and legislation from others undertaking the duties and responsibilities assigned to this particular professional group.
- The profession is usually held in high esteem and public respect, and its members commonly receive high financial rewards.

Students of a professional group must undertake a programme of study that enables them to develop the body of knowledge, skill, understanding and experience as well as to adopt the professional culture which sets the baseline for professional practice. However, at the point of registration, students become novice practitioners who are continually required to advance their competence in a particular field. When they move from one field to another, some of their skills may be transferable, but they may also lack some knowledge and skills that are required to maintain patients' safety and the quality of their care. Whenever someone moves to a new field of practice, there should always be a period of induction. Part of the induction process is to ensure students or new practitioners are competent and safe to practise (Slevin, 2003).

This chapter covers dimensions of professional practice and takes nursing as an example of a professional organizational group.

Activity

- Reflect on your own professional journey so far. Are you a new student to the profession or are you moving into a new field of practice that relates to the older person?
- Reflect on your attitudes now compared to your attitudes when you were new to the profession.
- Critically examine your thoughts and feelings as you face another part of your journey.
- Describe how competent you feel when working with older people
- Assess your knowledge and skills deficits.

BECOME A REGISTERED NURSE

Nursing became a registered profession regulated by an Act of Parliament in 1919, following 30 years of political activity on the part of concerned nurses. Their victory was recorded in an editorial published on 5 July 1919 by the then editor of the *British Journal of*

Nursing, Mrs Ethel Bedford Fenwick, who was one of the most militant and vocal nurses of the time. She described the achievement as 'placing in the forefront the registration of nurses, for the standardization and improvement of nursing education, for the protection of the sick and for the improvement of the economic status of trained nurses'. Professional regulation had come into being. Registered nurses must know and understand the Code of Professional Conduct and apply its principles to every part of daily professional practice.

Activity

You may wish to re-read the code now, before moving on to the discussion about what it means to be professional.

Being a registered nurse carries with it a range of responsibilities, which will be explored in detail later in this chapter. The professional register certifies three things about nurses whose names appear:

- They are able to practise according to professional protocols and codes.
- They possess the skills and knowledge necessary for effective practice.
- They possess a thorough understanding of the key influences that shape their professional practice.

MANAGEMENT OF REGISTRATION

For many years, regulation was managed by general nursing councils (GNCs), such as the GNC for England and Wales and the GNC for Scotland. In 1979 an Act of Parliament established the basis of the modern regulatory structure and led to the formation of the United Kingdom Central Council for Nursing, Midwifery and Health Visiting (UKCC) and the national boards. These bodies were themselves subject to review in 1998 and replaced by a single statutory body in 2002, called the Nursing and Midwifery Council (NMC). The powers of the NMC are set out in the *Nursing and Midwifery Order* 2001 (NMC, 2001). This new regulatory body is responsible for setting standards for the profession. It is also charged with maintaining a professional register that is instrumental in upholding public protection. The Nursing and Midwifery Council is currently the regulatory body for nursing, midwifery and health visiting throughout the UK. Its principal function is to set and improve standards of education, practice and conduct for the professions it regulates.

What does it mean to be a registered nurse?

All of the 650 000 nurses, midwives and health visitors whose names are currently on the register of the NMC have met the standards of the regulatory body. These standards relate to

- education
- registration
- continuing professional development and post-registration education practice (PREP)
- conduct.

The professional register lies at the heart of the Council's activity, which is focused on public protection. No one may practise as a nurse, midwife or health visitor in the UK without effective registration with the Council. The Council also sets requirements for pre-registration nursing programmes. Persons successfully completing one of these programmes are eligible for registration. Practitioners are required to renew their registration every three years.

Educational programmes

It is possible to take either a higher-education diploma or a degree course to qualify as a nurse. Education is provided by universities, with placements in local hospital and community settings. The course is 50% theory and 50% practice. The first year is a common foundation programme, which will introduce students to the basic principles of nursing. This is then followed by a further two years (total programme hours 4600), which specializes in adult, child, mental health or learning disability nursing. Full-time diploma courses last three years. Degree courses last three or four years.

Nursing professionals

'As a registered nurse, midwife or health visitor, you are personally accountable for your practice (NMC, 2002, p.1).' This quotation begins one of the most important documents on professional nursing practice, the *Code of Professional Conduct*, which will be examined in detail in this chapter. You also need to be aware of the *National Service Framework for Older People* (Department of Health, 2001), as it also considers professionalism in terms of general standards of care relating to older patients, based on the recommendations of *Better Care, Higher Standards: A Charter for Long-Term Care* (Department of Health, 1999). Here are some examples of what the standards ensure:

- Clean, dry sheets are provided by the NHS.
- Older people are given food and drink that meets proper standards and provides appropriate nutrition.
- Older people have the right and access to top-quality care.
- Mixed-sex wards are replaced by single-sex wards to foster proper standards of privacy and dignity for older people.
- Older people can remain independent for as long as possible.
- Older people will be consulted about their care.

NHS boards will have a duty of clinical governance to ensure that the standards are met. The standards will apply to all sectors: acute, nursing homes and residential and community care. If you work in Scotland, Wales or Northern Ireland, seek out equivalent standards, documents and policies that apply to your country.

CHARACTERISTICS OF A PROFESSION AND A NURSING PROFESSIONAL

Features and images of professionalism

What is professionalism in nursing? Does it mean becoming more like a doctor? Or is there some other notion of professionalism that's more applicable to nursing? Professional occupation can be described as having a systematic body of knowledge that is underpinned by evidence from research or practice, a code of professional practice, an altruistic nature and a legal framework of standards and obligations within which it operates. Figure 4.1 a health-care professional sharing a humorous moment with an older person.

Figure 4.1

Humour in care

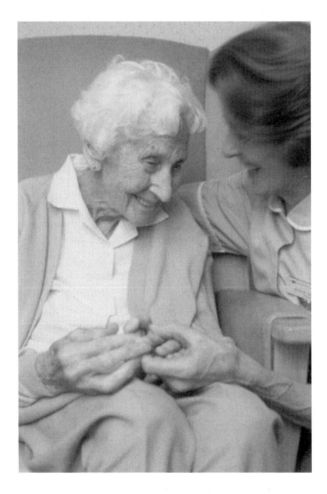

Activity

Read widely about professional characteristics. Write in your journal the various characteristics described for professional practice.

Different contributors to the debate about professionalism emphasize different aspects. Some people consider that a body of knowledge is less important than the profession's level of autonomy and control over itself (Elston, 1991). Others equate the professionalization of nursing with a drive to change the image of nursing, both in the eyes of its members and those of the general public. The image of nurses as handmaidens to doctors has been widely promoted in popular films and television programmes over the past 30 years. Florence Nightingale reportedly insisted that the doctor took decisions about who should be patients and what should be done for them, the nurse's function being to assist the doctor (Porter, 1990).

Feminist perspectives on medicine and nursing have recently suggested that these professions are viewed in a predominantly masculine way, reflecting the masculine view of the world that permeates society as a whole: 'being detached and calmly evaluating the options, being strictly in control of self and, indeed, of others' (Davies, 1996a). In the second of her two articles, Davies (1996b) argues for a new image of professionalism for nursing, one that reflects commitment rather than detachment, and which emphasizes the group rather than the individual. She provides a set of contrasting features for what she sees as the 'old professionalism' and the 'new professionalism'. According to Davies, changes in approaches to health care over recent years reflect new professionalism: nurses taking on the role of patient advocate, empowerment of patients, and other forms of user participation. She urges an approach that enables the professional to value qualities other than the scientific and abstract, and acknowledges the intuitive aspects of nursing and the importance of experience.

Schön (1992) has argued that a professional approach is one where the professional appreciates that the problems he or she face contain uncertainties. It involves a willingness to learn together with the patient. We judge people as professional in terms of how they think about their work; Schön calls this 'reflection in action'. You may realize that the terms 'profession' and 'professional' are used in a variety of ways according to the context or purposes of the user. They are not absolute terms. When people use these words, they often assume that others will have the same image of 'profession' or 'professional' as they do themselves. These assumptions can be misleading. In health care, professionalism can be seen as the pursuit of humanitarian goals in which the interests of patients outweigh concern with professional status. Patients are kept well informed and given an autonomous say in their treatment. This type of relationship between professional and patient is characterized by mutual consensus and trust.

Activity

- Reflect on Mary's experience and examine whether the qualities just outlined form part of Mary's experience of professionals during her outpatient visits.
- Explore the concept of professionalism in greater depth.
- Look at popular images of health-care professionals in the media, and the influence of politics.
- Identify the media's portrayal of various professional groups.

Care, caring, cure and health

What are the meanings of terms such as 'health', 'cure' and 'care'? This is important because meanings contain assumptions about the health care of older patients. Analysing the meanings can help you to

- recognize your values;
- consider how your values relate to your everyday practice of caring for older patients;
- reflect on whether your values complement the values in your workplace, the local community and the national scene.

The Health Advisory Service 2000 report *Not Because They Are Old* (Health Advisory Service 2000, 1998) stated, among other things, that patients, their relatives and staff must all take responsibility for challenging negative views about old age and the propensity for ill health, particularly the belief that prospects for recovery are gloomy.

Care and caring

You may have entered nursing because you wanted to care for people who are sick, ill, wounded, incapacitated, disabled or old. You know that many people need care when they are older and you may assume that caring is a fundamental human quality. But perhaps it is not that simple. Caring can mean different things to different people. It can be a divisive term; for example, how can you care for someone who refuses care but who also needs it? How does the concept of caring relate to ideas of justice, free will, choice, generosity and faithfulness? Caring can involve the notion of empowerment. To empower their older patients, nurses need to consider where their own strengths lie and develop the personal qualities that make intimacy possible between themselves and their patients (Clarke, 1991). These qualities are the basis for reflective practice in health care (Johns, 1996). Here are some views of others involved in caring for older people:

- I wanted to go into palliative care of older patients because it seemed to me that caring for others is at the heart of the job. No other nursing would offer me the same opportunity to provide care.
- I look after my father who is almost totally dependent now. I feel guilty when I take a week off to go on holiday, because it looks as if I don't really care about him.

- I went into care of older people, to be honest, because I thought it would be easier for me, going back after such a long break from nursing, than working in an acute ward.

Cure

The meaning of 'cure' relates to the successful outcome of a process that aims to correct a problem. People are cured because they are ill. But in reality the outcomes are rarely one hundred per cent successful. There are many gradations in the language of medical intervention, including the concepts of remission and side effects. The moral absolutism inherent in the concept of cure is signalled by use of the same words in many religious belief systems:

- There is no health in us.
- We seek remission from sins.
- Repentance is a cure for souls.

Health

In its constitution of 1946 the World Health Organization (WHO) first defined health as 'a state of complete physical, mental, and social well-being and not merely the absence of disease or infirmity'. In 1978 WHO stated: 'Health ... is a fundamental human right' (WHO, 1978). In 1984 WHO altered its original definition of health to: 'The extent to which an individual or group is able, on the one hand, to realise aspirations and satisfy needs, and, on the other hand, to change or cope with the environment. Health is, therefore, a resource for everyday life, not an object of living; it is a positive concept emphasizing social and personal resources, as well as physical capabilities' (WHO, 1984).

Consider the following exchange between a daughter and her 70-year-old mother, overheard in Lancashire. How do they differ in their concepts of sickness and health?

DAUGHTER: It's a shame about Mrs Butler.
MOTHER: She's not as sick as me, you know.
DAUGHTER: Mother, she's died.
MOTHER: Well, she weren't as sick as me.

Does ageism exist in nursing?

Ageism is covered more generally in Chapter 2 and here we consider it from a professional standpoint; it may help your learning to refer back and forth between here and Chapter 2. Wade (1996) considers that one of the greatest threats to a person's self-esteem lies in how they are seen by others. Negative images and stereotypical thinking about growing old do exist among professionals. These include views of older people as inflexible, dependent individuals who suffer from poor health, mental frailty and social isolation. Consider how the media often portray the older person, as in the following extract from 'The Granny Spy Scandal' (*Sunday Mirror*, 12 September 1999):

> '*I'm 87, my memory is not what it was, but I have no regrets ... I spied to save Russia from defeat.*'
>
> *Melita Norwood looked every inch the great granny when she came out from her end-of-terrace house and shuffled down the garden path. Her thinning, silver-grey hair was side-parted and clipped back. Petite, bespectacled and almost lost in her A-line grey skirt and old-fashioned, floppy-collared floral print blouse, she wouldn't have looked out of place in a post office queue waiting to pick up her pension.*

Negative images of the old and the ageing are thought to result in the stigmatization and marginalization of older people (Victor, 1999). According to Littler (1997), 'An individual age is more than just a number. It becomes the focus of certain social norms, values and behaviour patterns seen as appropriate for a particular chronological age'. Littler argues that society imposes on the individual a relatively clear set of expectations and restrictions. Blytheway (1995) states that ageism generates and reinforces a fear of growing old as well as producing barriers to resources and opportunities which others enjoy. Health professionals who work with older people are often more ageist than the general public because there is an assumption that the problems experienced by their patients are common to all old people (Redfern, 1991).

This Bed My Centre is the diary of Ellen Newton, born in Melbourne, Australia, in 1896. She worked for many years as a freelance writer, broadcaster and short story writer, and in various libraries and bookshops. In her seventies, suffering from angina, Ellen spent six years in a series of nursing homes. She recorded those years in her secret diary. At age 81 she rebelled. Being of sound mind, she discharged herself from hospital and, with help from her family, found a small flat where she lived happily for many years, preparing her diary for publication and writing her first novel.

THE CODE OF PROFESSIONAL CONDUCT

The NMC, which replaced the UKCC on 1 April 2002, has published the new code of professional conduct. The new code which took effect in June 2002 was jointly agreed by the UKCC and the NMC, and combined three important publications: the *Scope of Professional Practice* (UKCC, 1992b), *Guidelines for Professional Practice* (UKCC, 1996a), and the current *Code of Professional Conduct* (UKCC, 2002). It was decided that one document was less extensive than three, hence it would be more useful and informative.

The Code of Professional Conduct is the shared values of all UK regulatory bodies and states that all registered nurses and midwives should

- respect all patients and clients as individuals;
- obtain consent before giving any treatment or care;

- protect confidential information;
- cooperate with others in a team;
- maintain your professional knowledge and competence;
- be trustworthy;
- act to identify and minimize risks to patients and clients.

The NMC intends to keep this code under continual review and welcomes any comments from practitioners and members of the public.

Background

What is the Code of Professional Conduct? It is not a piece of legislation but it grew out of the legislative requirement to 'provide in such a manner as it thinks fit, advice for nurses, midwives and health visitors on standards of professional conduct' (UKCC, 1992a). It therefore has its basis in the law and is the template against which your behaviour would be judged if you were ever to be called to account for your practice. Such judgement could be through a local disciplinary hearing in your workplace or, in extreme circumstances, in front of the NMC's professional conduct committee. The code also offers the public a description of what can be expected of registered nurses, an essential part of the openness and visibility increasingly required by the professions if they are to have public confidence.

Key elements: your responsibility

If you do not already have your own copy of the code, obtain one straight away from the NMC, 23 Portland Place, London W1N 4JT or from the NMC website at www.nmc-uk.org. It is free and you really do need one of your own. Make sure you have the current edition.

The Code of Professional Conduct

Is the Code of Professional Conduct at the heart of your practice, something you think about every day and use regularly? Or is it something you see as irrelevant to the real day-to-day work of nursing older patients? Perhaps a bit of both? This part looks at how the code can be used to support good practice, as the basis from which to challenge unacceptable standards of care, and to offer a realistic framework within which awkward dilemmas can be considered.

The code is an essential adjunct to care, particularly in the field of nursing older patients where there are many ethical and moral dilemmas to consider. Perhaps the most important part of the code is the stem: 'As a registered nurse, midwife or health visitor, you are personally accountable for your practice and, in the exercise of your professional accountability, must: ...'. Seven individual clauses then follow, each identifying a specific aspect of your professional responsibility. Each clause is expanded in the code to give a fuller description of your responsibilities. Remember that each separate clause arises from that stem. Look at it again. It is unequivocal; indeed it may even make quite uncomfortable reading. As a registered nurse, you are personally accountable for your practice. This really means *you*, not anyone else, not a senior member of staff, a doctor or another health-care professional. Saying 'but she told me to do it' is never a justification for poor practice.

It makes you think hard, doesn't it? And it may be very different from the way a lot of nurses were originally taught, when it was very clear who gave the orders and who obeyed them. Now you cannot blame anyone else; you are responsible. People who use health-care services increasingly expect that those caring for them should offer a choice of informed care which is based on the best evidence available, and which also involves the individuals concerned in making decisions about their own care. And in terms of professional worth, it is much more satisfying to know that you are doing the best that can be done. The other part of the stem to look at is the last part: 'As a registered nurse ... you ... must ...' . Again, there is no polite option, this is what you *must* do, not what you may do, or would like to do, or might do some days but not others. This is a really challenging imperative and one that does get challenged (Vousden, 1998). Now let's look closely at each of the seven clauses.

Respect
As a registered nurse or midwife you should respect all patients and clients as individuals.

This clause states how a nurse or midwife should recognize and respect all aspects of patient and client care.

Consent
As a registered nurse or midwife you should obtain consent before giving treatment or care. This clause expands to state that all patients and clients are entitled to receive and understand information about their condition and treatment and therefore have a right to refuse health-care intervention. Before any treatment or care is given, valid consent must be sought from the patient or legal guardian or someone who is legally competent. Information given must be accurate and truthful and presented so that it will be understood.

Team cooperation
As a registered nurse or midwife you must cooperate with others in the team. Here 'team' means patient, client, families, carers, health and social care professionals in the NHS, independent and voluntary sectors. There is also an explanation of how to work cooperatively in a team. Figure 4.2 shows a multidisciplinary team providing care.

Confidentiality
As a registered nurse or midwife you should protect confidential information. All patient or client information is confidential and should be used solely for the purpose that it was given. It should be made clear to patients or clients that it would be impractical to obtain consent on

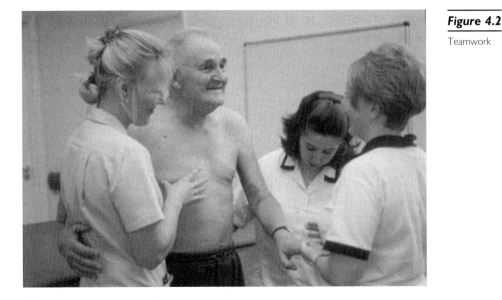

Figure 4.2

Teamwork

every occasion that another member of the care team required some information on the individual, so information may be made available to other members of the team delivering care to the individual. If consent cannot be sought then disclosure of information outside the care team may only take place if it is in the public's interest (when protection is required for the individual or another party if there is a risk of significant harm) or they are required by an order of the court or by law. If there is an issue of child protection, it is essential that national and local policies are adhered to.

Knowledge and competence

As a registered nurse or midwife you should maintain your professional knowledge and competence. Your knowledge and skills must be kept up to date throughout your working life. To practise competently you must possess the knowledge, skills and abilities required for lawful, safe and effective practice without direct supervision.

The implication is that professional practice never stays still. All registered practitioners need to

- review their practice regularly;
- extend their own knowledge base;
- look for ways of improving the care they give.

This is partly what post-registration education practice (PREP) is about, but it goes far beyond the minimum required by the legislation. When you consider expanding your practice somehow, you must be certain that you have the knowledge, skills and abilities to do the new work. Merely having a long-standing desire to do heart surgery doesn't equip you to perform it. So if, in the interests of improving older patient care, you or a colleague would like to do something different, you may need to be shown what to do and how to do it by a more experienced practitioner. This could include

- learning from someone in another health-care profession;
- searching the literature;
- undertaking a relevant course.

Trustworthy

As a registered nurse or midwife you must be trustworthy. The code describes that a registered nurse or midwife must behave in a way that upholds the reputation of the profession. Any behaviour that compromises this reputation may call registration into question, even when not directly related. Refusal must be given to any gifts, favours or hospitality that may at a later date be seen as a way to obtain preferential treatment.

Minimize risks

As a registered nurse or midwife you must act to identify and minimize risks to patients and clients. This obligation means that all members of the team should work together to promote health-care environments that are conducive to safe, therapeutic and ethical practice. You should act quickly to protect patients or clients if you believe a colleague is unfit to work for reasons of health, conduct or competence. Awareness of current legislation on the protection for people who raise concerns about health and safety issues must be up to date.

Facts and figures

One of the most effective ways of judging the quality of professional care is to examine that profession's professional conduct or disciplinary records. Allegations of misconduct in nursing are made to the NMC. Is there anything that an investigation of the statistics can tell us about care in this sector? Regrettably, the picture is not good. The two most common offences that come before the NMC's professional conduct machinery and reported in the *Professional Conduct Annual Report 2002–2003* (NMC, 2003) are issues of clinical practice, including failing to keep accurate records, and physical or verbal abuse of older patients.

Most complaints come from employers (40%), usually in association with disciplinary proceedings at the workplace. The NMC also receives complaints from the police as it is required to inform the regulatory body when a registered practitioner is convicted of a criminal offence, even in cases of minor matters that are unlikely to lead to any further action. Finally, complaints are also made by the public, colleagues, supervisors of midwives, the National Care Standards Commission and others.

Staff development and caring for older patients
Studies that took place in certain hospitals (UKCC, 1997; Health Advisory Service 2000, 1998) show that within older patient care there is a need for

- compulsory induction and preceptorship programmes;
- improved systems for continuing professional development, of which PREP (see below) is an integral part;
- wider access to development opportunities;
- clinical supervision;
- staff appraisal that identifies education and training needs of staff;
- opportunities for multiprofessional education before and after registration;
- the development of teaching nursing homes, although the different models of teaching nursing homes would need to be explored and the most appropriate model selected;
- further development of work-based learning, open learning and distance learning.

PREP

The NMC's standards for continuing professional development are known as the PREP requirements (UKCC, 1995). Since 1995 they require registered nurses, midwives and health visitors to

- complete a minimum of five days of study activity every three years;
- keep a personal professional profile;
- undertake a statutory return-to-practice programme after a break of five years or more.

These standards are significant in that for the first time all practitioners on the NMC's register are required to take steps to maintain and develop their knowledge and competence; before 1995 this was a statutory requirement for midwives only.

Clinical governance

Clinical governance is discussed in Chapter 3. This section looks at its relevance to professional obligation and responsibility. In response to numerous service failures, particularly to the old, the cognitively challenged and the very young, the government has implemented a framework of clinical governance. The principal aim was to assure quality and that care is given by professionals who are competent to practise using contemporary scientific evidence. This requires that each individual practitioner must continue their learning throughout the life of their professional practice. Maintaining skills for lifelong learning is now essential for professional practice. Lifelong learning skills are also required when transferring nursing skills to work in different settings, when learning new skills to meet new service demands, or when adapting to new technology or new scientific evidence. The Department of Health (2001, p. 1) suggests that

> *lifelong learning is about growth and opportunity, about making sure that our staff, the teams and organisations they relate to, and work in, can acquire new knowledge and skills both to realise their potential and help shape and change things for the better.*

Basford and Slevin (2003) have identified that the government hopes to ensure that lifelong learning is entrenched within continuing professional development and the demonstration of each individual practitioner's competence to practise. Moreover, there are some underpinning core values which relate to lifelong learning that will enable each practitioner to work within the notion of quality and proficiency. All learning, formal or informal, will be recognized and valued and recorded in a professional portfolio. It is suggested that lifelong learning principles will enable learners to be

- innovative in their practice;
- flexible and responsive to changing demands;
- resourceful in their methods of working;
- able to work as change agents;
- able to share good practice and knowledge;
- adaptable to changing health-care needs;
- challenging and creative in their practice;
- self-reliant in their way of working;
- responsible and accountable for their work.

Activity

- Describe the difference between a learning portfolio and a professional portfolio.
- Identify the skills required for lifelong learning in a knowledge society.
- Discuss these issues with your peers.
- Discuss how Mary's experience could have been improved if the professionals working with Mary had skills to advance their knowledge through lifelong learning concepts.

Research and development

Under clinical governance, organizations need to establish systems to help nurses use scientific evidence by enabling them to

- obtain information and evidence;
- implement good practice based on scientific evidence;
- monitor the effects of their practice;
- disseminate the results;
- critically review the evidence as applied to their field of practice.

Organizations also need to make sure staff are supported and supervised to maximize quality and effectiveness.

Audit

Audit is about setting and using local, national and international standards and guidelines on effectiveness and quality of treatment and interventions. This chapter covers many of the issues involved in professional practice. However, there is always more to learn, as practice develops to reflect continuing technological, clinical, social, political and demographic changes. By continuing your learning throughout your practice, you and your older patients will benefit. Use the internet to help keep abreast of developments.

OTHER CODES AFFECT SERVICE PROVISION TO OLDER PEOPLE

As a member of a care team you will work with members of other professions. Among these team members will be doctors and social workers. Each of these groups has professional principles that guide and govern their activities.

General Medical Council

The public trust doctors to set and monitor their own professional standards. In return, doctors must give their patients high-quality medical care. The legal authority of the General Medical Council (GMC) is the Medical Act 1983, which gives powers to protect, promote and maintain the health and safety of the public. The GMC maintains a registry of doctors. Whenever a doctor fails to meet professional standards, the GMC acts to protect patients from harm, if necessary, by striking doctors off the register and removing their right to practise medicine. The GMC has strong and effective legal powers designed to maintain the standards the public have a right to expect of doctors. The GMC exists to protect patients; the interests of the medical profession are protected by other organizations.

Duties of a doctor

Patients must be able to trust doctors with their lives and well-being. To justify that trust, the GMC defines what a profession must do to maintain a good standard of practice and care and to show respect for human life. According to the GMC website (www.gmc-uk.org), a doctor must

- make the care of a patient one's first concern;
- treat every patient politely and considerately;
- respect patients' dignity and privacy;
- listen to patients and respect their views;
- give patients information in a way they can understand;
- respect the rights of patients to be fully involved in decisions about their care;
- keep professional knowledge and skills up to date;

- recognize the limits of one's own professional competence;
- be honest and trustworthy;
- respect and protect confidential information;
- make sure that one's personal beliefs do not prejudice a patient's care;
- act quickly to protect patients from risk if there is good reason to believe that oneself or a colleague may not be fit to practise;
- avoid abusing one's position as a doctor;
- work with colleagues in the ways that best serve patients' interests.

General Social Care Council

The General Social Care Council (GSCC) was established on 1 October 2001 under the legal framework of the Care Standards Act 2000 (Department of Health, 2000). The GSCC covers England; equivalent bodies cover Scotland, Northern Ireland and Wales. The GSCC is the guardian of standards for the social care workforce with the aim of increasing the protection of service users, their carers and the general public. The GSCC has three key functions. First, it establishes codes of conduct and practice for social care workers. Second, it regulates the profession and supports training and education so that social care workers will know what is expected of them and the public will know the standards they can expect through the codes of conduct. Finally, it registers the social care workforce in England.

Social work is a professional activity. Social workers also have obligations to service users, to their employers, to one another, to colleagues in other disciplines and to society. Social workers attempt to relieve and prevent hardship and suffering. They have a responsibility to help individuals, families, groups and communities through the provision and operation of appropriate services as well as by contributing to social planning. Their work may include, but is not limited to, interpersonal practice, group work, community work, social development, social action, policy development, research, social work education, and supervisory and managerial functions in these fields.

Social work is committed to five basic values:

- human dignity and worth
- social justice
- service to humanity
- integrity
- competence.

Codes of practice for social care workers and employers

The first UK-wide codes of practice for social care workers and employers were launched in September 2002 (GSCC, 2002). They provide a clear guide for all those who work in social care, setting out the standards of practice and conduct that should be met by workers and their employers. They build on existing good practice and the shared values of the sector. The codes are a critical part of regulating the social care workforce and helping to improve levels of professionalism and public protection. They were developed following extensive consultation with social care workers, service users and carers in 2002. There is a code of conduct that all social care workers will be expected to follow to ensure they meet agreed standards on conduct and practice, and also a code of practice that all employers in social care will be expected to follow to ensure they know the standards they should meet to enable workers to do their jobs well. Many people rely on the honesty, integrity and professional skills of social care workers, and these codes set out the standards people can expect of them. You can see the details of this code by going to the GSCC website at www.gscc.org.uk.

Social Care Registry

The GSCC and the other social care regulatory councils around the UK began the process of registration in April 2003, starting with qualified social workers. Registration of the social care workforce was introduced by law to increase protection for the people who use social care services and their carers. Social care workers of all levels will be registered, from care workers through to directors of social services. England has the GSCC. Scotland, Northern Ireland and Wales each have an equivalent body that maintains its own list:

- Care Council for Wales
- Northern Ireland Social Care Council
- Scottish Social Services Council.

Registration of the social care workforce is well under way, with thousands of qualified social workers currently filling in their applications.

Global standards

Across the world, countries have established standards of practice and codes of ethics for health-care professionals, and the UK is one of the leaders. Through international organizations such as the United Nations, all countries are encouraged to set high standards and to work towards common elements in their standards. These developments benefit health-care workers seeking employment in other countries as well as the public, who are increasingly mobile on a global scale.

Activity ────────────────────────────

- Take the codes for other team members described earlier and consider how they are similar to the NMC's Code of Professional Conduct.
- How does each professional code relate to professional knowledge and competence?
- What do they say about patient and client rights?
- What value does the public receive from the registration of nurses, doctors and social workers?

- As you become more familiar with the implications of having your own code, find opportunities to talk with other professionals about their registration requirements and professional standards.

ROLES AND SKILLS FOR WORKING EFFECTIVELY WITH OLDER PEOPLE

Nursing is an ancient occupation, but the capabilities needed by an effective nurse are still being debated today. There are many different ideologies of nursing within the profession itself and among other groups such as doctors and the general public. This diversity can be beneficial, because it makes us question what we mean by 'the nursing profession'. During the process of questioning we must continually justify our professional existence. The NMC Code of Professional Conduct explains that serious failure to meet its standards can result in removal of a nurse's name from the register, thereby prohibiting them from practice. That is because there are some basic, and apparently enduring, areas of agreement about what a nurse should be and how a nurse should behave.

The helping role

Nurses perform their role because people need the particular kind of help they are trained to offer. They play a helping role in the sense that helping others is integral to what they do. Nurses work in organizations dedicated to meeting the needs of patients. Everything that is done there contributes, directly or indirectly, to this end. All their professional interactions with colleagues and others feed in one way or another into their helping role.

Why do people help?

A characteristic of helping patients is that the focus of attention is on the patient being helped, rather than on the helper. As a nurse, the needs of your patients come first. The professional role requires you to act in whatever way brings most health benefit to them. Put this way, the helping role can appear selfless. It would probably give a fuller picture if you consider some of the reasons people take on a helping role – why they care – for a living. They may want to

- help alleviate suffering;
- give something to society and the community;
- gain a sense of personal satisfaction;
- feel useful, valued, needed and/or appreciated by others.

They may also feel a strong sense of responsibility, or be attracted by the dramatic side of being involved in life-or-death situations. They may be following a family tradition, imitating a model they admire or satisfying a deep-seated impulse. There may be all kinds of factors, conscious and unconscious, behind the choice of a helping role.

Empathy with older patients

Nurses do not have a monopoly on caring and empathy. Other professional roles also require empathy to a high degree. But what is empathy? It is usually explained as a way in which one person perceives and understands the experience of another. It is closely related to intuition, but it can be more consciously developed than intuition, which is seen as innate. Empathy can involve leaving one's own subjective experience and entering that of another person (Rogers, 1961). Figure 4.3 shows a health-care professional demonstrating empathy.

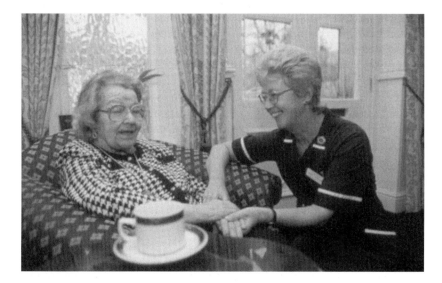

Figure 4.3

Empathetic approaches in care

Do nurses need empathy with their older patients?

What value does empathy have? People can learn about each other's thoughts through observation or discussion, but thoughts on their own do not convey the character of another person's inner life; their feelings and sense of being are important too. Amid the pressures of a working day, carers may forget that each individual is unique. It can be easy for nurses to fall into the habit of generalizing and making assumptions about all older patients. Cultivating empathy is one way to counter the depersonalizing atmosphere of many health-care environments. It has been suggested that empathy can be developed into a specialized communication skill to gain information not usually available through ordinary rational techniques. This may be an important dimension of caring, although it may be inappropriate in curing, where objectivity and rational judgement could be hindered by emotions.

Here are three extracts from Ellen Newton's nursing home diary (Newton, 1980):

> *Last night was strangely peaceful. Five hours' good sleep. Yet today, nothing is on time. Linen is in more than usual short supply, more strangers on the staff, and two unruly patients close to my door. They*

sound as if they are not just ill. Part of the clamour could be unhappiness and insecurity. . . .

Matron is leaving. For several weeks she has not been quite with us – some involvement we know nothing about. She tells me she will stay here until a new matron is forthcoming. It will be hard to find someone to measure up to her. We shouldn't expect to harness her quality to this kind of 'hospital' where the outcome of every case must always be the same. She needs the challenge of fighting to save lives. I think she would probably enjoy a refresher course in new nursing trends, too. For this enclosed collection of old ladies, and two or three men – it is in no way a community – her going will be a far bigger upheaval than any change of government in the world outside. Here nothing ever happens that is at all unexpected, unless it is traumatic. 'Stop thinking about yourself.' . . .

The last few weeks we have had a full-time charge sister. Young, not so very experienced, but very well trained. She's pleasant, compassionate, quick-thinking and most dependable. It is good, after all the recent stopping and starting, to have someone like her around.

Research in the context of care for older patients with Alzheimer's disease has shown that a vital feature of caregiving is the way in which it can lend meaning to difficult tasks. Nurses and other carers often gain personal strength when they find meaning in the care they give. And the person receiving care seems more likely to respond positively if the carer finds their task meaningful.

Effective caring also seems to require that the carer provides those cared for with real choice. In caring for older patients, this might involve restoring rights and freedoms to choose to live the way they wish to (Tones and Tilford, 1994). This view is emphasized by one of the key recommendations in *Not Because They are Old* (Health Advisory Service 2000, 1998) that older people and their families must be more involved with their care at every stage and in relation to every decision. You may be interested to read Lancely's work on the controlling language used by nurses with older patients (Lancely, 1985). Reporting on a study that analysed the content of nurses' interactions with frail older patients, it shows how the nurses' interactions often prevented patients from taking a full part in their care.

The caring relationship demands of the carer a willingness to forgo, as far as possible, any core status and authority. This position does not demean the knowledge and skills of health-care professionals. In fact, it takes special skills and professionalism to promote choice, trust and other features that make it possible to create a caring relationship.

Activity

- Look at *Values and the Person: Ideas that Influence Health Care*, one of the modules from the BSc in professional practice pathway (Macmillan Magazines, 1997), for more about caring, and about empathy as a therapeutic intervention. See also *Influences in Health Care: Media Perspectives* (Macmillan Open Learning, 1997).

EMPOWERING NURSING HOME RESIDENTS

In one study, a group of nursing home residents was given the opportunity to influence how the home was run (e.g. by choosing menus) and to take some responsibilities. They were encouraged to arrange the furniture in their rooms and given potted plants to care for. A control group of residents occupying a different but similar floor in the home were also given potted plants, but were told that the nursing staff would look after them. Measures of activity levels and general happiness of the two groups revealed that the 'responsibility' group were more alert, active and contented than their counterparts. A year and a half later the experimental group had (i) maintained their quality of life and (ii) the death rate of the empowered group was half the death rate of residents who lacked the benefits of actual and perceived control over their lives (Tones and Tilford, 1994).

Your expectations of older patients

The nature of the nursing help often needs to change and this can affect the satisfaction experienced by nurses. The large number of support workers found in the care of older patients may be a cause for concern. Those aspects of health care that are often assumed to be the domain of untrained support workers could be the very aspects that many nurses feel make nursing worthwhile.

The continuing care of older people

In 1994 the UKCC established a group to address concerns about the nursing and health-visiting contribution to the continuing care of older people. The group considered the ways in which older people gain access to care in institutional and non-institutional settings. The aims of the group were to promote and maintain maximum potential for self-care. To this end, the group identified four areas in which nursing and health visiting can make a positive contribution to continuing care of older patients (UKCC, 1997).

Specialist practice skills and knowledge

The older person who has access to specialist nurses and health visitors is more knowledgeable, more proficient in self-care and more satisfied with the care received. Teams could be led by nurses and health visitors whereas other patients, such as those in residential homes, could also benefit from easy access to specialist district nursing, health visiting and practice nursing skills. There is the potential and the need to develop in the nursing home sector a model similar to that used in teaching hospitals. These 'teaching nursing homes' would be centres of academic and practical excellence and would provide students with placements in clinical practice before and after registration. This concept originated in the US and there is now a large body of literature describing nurse-led models and other models for teaching nursing homes.

Activity

Search for articles on teaching nursing homes by Brendan McCormack at the Royal College of Nursing and Professor David Challis at the University of Manchester. You could also search the internet for information about teaching nursing homes.

Assessment and review of needs

Nurses and health visitors should play a crucial role in the assessment and review of older patients' day-to-day care needs. They can offer a holistic perspective on assessment and the meeting of individual, family and community needs. Assessment tools must reflect the nursing and health-visiting care required.

Health promotion and maintenance

Health promotion in the continuing care of older people is sometimes undervalued and unrecognized, and not just by busy nurses, so many of whom often have insufficient time for all but the core responsibilities. Promoting health and preventing ill health can be managed as a major nursing and health-visiting priority, particularly in continuing care, where improved fitness can minimize illness, disability and dependency.

Working in partnership with patients and carers

Continuing care is enhanced by partnerships between those who provide care. Nurses and health visitors have a crucial role to play in promoting this partnership approach. They could act as advocates to support self-care and autonomy for older people. A good working relationship among nurses, health visitors, other carers and older people promotes informed decision making and patient autonomy. *United They Stand* (Audit Commission, 1995) identified several aspects of health care that contribute to providing effective continuing care:

- education, induction and clinical supervision
- an organizational culture committed to continuing care
- positive attitudes of nurses towards older people
- supportive and committed management
- respect for the contribution of other members of the care team
- appropriate delegation and supervision.

Activity

- Spend time considering aspects of health care and their meaning in practice. If possible, try to think of a practical example of something that would improve the continuing care of older people.

- Read *The Coming of Age: Improving Care Services for Older People* (Audit Commission, 1997).
- Use your learning diary to record your personal reflections in and on your practice.

Professional accountability

Midwives, health visitors and nurses' demands for increased professional recognition bring with them increased responsibilities. Whereas once doctors were assumed to have overall responsibility for the treatment of patients, now nurses increasingly make independent decisions on nursing care for which they are legally accountable in a court of law. Many older patients too are becoming aware of their power to litigate if things go wrong, and they are able to sue individual professionals as well as health trusts or other authorities. You need to know the law as it affects you and your practice; ignorance of the law is no defence. You are a professional and it is assumed that you know your legal position so that you carry out your practice in a way that is not criminal and that affords adequate protection to your patients and colleagues.

What is accountability?

The principle of accountability in nursing comes from the Code of Professional Conduct and various laws, particularly the common law of negligence (NMC, 2002). If you are put in charge of a task, as a professional, you can be 'called to account' for the consequences, especially if something goes wrong. If you perform a task, such as admitting a patient, you take responsibility for that task and its outcomes. Similarly, if you are supervising a student or team member, you take some responsibility for the individual's performance of the task; you can be called to account for some aspects of it. Here are two definitions from Pennels (1997):

- Accountability arises from a patient's reasonable expectation that, by virtue of their training and professional position, the nurse will be answerable to the patient while she or he is in the nurse's care. This is supported by the notion of negligence.
- Accountability is the requirement that each nurse is answerable and responsible for the outcome of his or her professional actions.

Delegating tasks to others

Much of the hands-on care of older people is delivered by care assistants. You, as a registered nurse, need to know how you are accountable when you delegate tasks to others. When delegating, you should ensure that you are aware of the established mix of skills in your team. 'Make sure that the person who does the work is able to do it and that appropriate levels of supervision or support are in place' (UKCC, 1996b). Complex legal matters can arise from delegating to other care workers and supporting other care workers. For guidelines, contact the Royal College of Nursing (www.rcn.org.uk) or Unison (www.unison.org.uk).

A paediatric model of delegation

Delegation of care to other family members takes place in children's wards and may provide a model for the care of older patients. Paediatric nursing is based on an ethos of family-centred care. The child is part of a family that continues to care for them when they are in hospital; this is vital for continuity of care when the child returns home. The sharing of care between nurses and family members needs to be negotiated with each family member. Different parents or carers have different strengths, and the nurse must establish what the parent or carer feels able to contribute.

In some wards, the named nurse has a negotiated arrangement with a named person about what tasks that person is able to do when in the ward with the children, including feeding and toileting. When the named person arrives in the ward, the nurse should always ask whether or not that person is opting into care. Some days the parent or carer may be exhausted or may be accompanied by a brother or sister and may not feel able to undertake care. It is important that the nurse establishes who is doing what.

Although each individual may be an independent and accountable practitioner, they also work as part of a team. Each team has members who have their own standards. In addition, the team develops standards of care, and these standards affect the client. The team is also affected by organizational and professional standards. Applying individual standards to health care can be problematic, because one person's standards may not be acceptable to others.

Activity

Write an account of how you are accountable. Reflect on your account after studying the following extract (NMC, 2002):

You are accountable to:
- *Your patients, through a duty of care, underpinned by a common-law duty to promote safety and efficiency, and legal responsibility through civil law;*
- *Your employer, as defined by the contract of employment and job description;*
- *Your profession, as stated in the relevant codes of conduct; and,*
- *The public.*

Accountable to the profession

The Code of Professional Conduct sets out the position on your accountability to the profession. You should know exactly what it says about your accountability in order to think clearly about your own ethical issues.

Accountable to your employer

Everyone has a contract of employment; UK law stipulates that all workers must be issued with a written contract of employment within

13 weeks of starting a job. Here are three things your contract could include:

- what was agreed at your interview
- any document which you have signed
- any implied terms of your employment.

The implied terms are those that may not have been discussed but which the court could assume to exist unless there is evidence to the contrary. For example, it is an implied term of a contract of employment that an employee will obey the reasonable instructions of the employer and will use all care and skill.

If you do something that contravenes this, perhaps by being grossly negligent, the employer can take disciplinary action against you for breach of your contract. The disciplinary action can include oral or written warnings, demotion, suspension and dismissal from your post. If you feel you have been unfairly dismissed, you can apply to an industrial tribunal for a hearing of unfair dismissal. If you are unclear about the policies and practices of your employer, you need to find out about them. Find out your organization's written or unwritten policies and procedures on dismissal, equal opportunities and discrimination, health and safety, and handling of hazardous materials. Is there a standard dismissals procedure and when was it last updated?

Autonomy

The UKCC report *Project 2000: A New Preparation for Practice* (UKCC, 1986) explained that autonomous practitioners were to exercise increasing clinical discretion and take on greater professional responsibility by taking their own decisions. They were also required to carry out more direct care, research, management, policy making and strategy development. Many nurses have autonomous practice as a professional aspiration. That is, you and your fellow professionals, not just your employer, make the decisions about your practice. You have your own caseload, perhaps working in a nurse-led unit. You and your unit admit and assess patients, perform all the caring during their stay and take responsibility for discharging them. In the past few years, health trusts and many nursing homes and community settings have taken a more managerial approach to running local health services; they take responsibility for the quality of their service and the costs. There is a clear link between responsibility and autonomy. If we wish to be autonomous, we then take responsibility for our decisions and the results of our actions.

THE ISSUES WHEN CARING FOR OLDER PERSONS

Authors such as Wade and Waters (1995) argue that by according low value and status to nurses who care for older people we perpetuate the undervaluing of older people. The problem is compounded by reduced technological, surgical and varied medical interventions associated with the care of older patients. Within the past decade, rapid expansion of the independent sector within this care group has produced further marginalization and demarcations. Barriers appear to separate care in the state sector and the independent sector (Nazarko, 1998). Attitudes towards older people and the fears and anxieties often held by health-care workers and the general public must therefore continue to be challenged. Heath (1998) has put forward a strong argument in support of changing attitudes towards care of the elderly. She believes this area of nursing care has already attracted 'visionary, articulate and pioneering nurses'. However, it will take much more work to overcome the belief that nursing the older person consists of no more than providing basic care, as expressed by one nurse returner we interviewed while developing this material: 'I decided to work in elderly care because I'd had four years out bringing up my kids and it was an easy option'.

The following quotation is about a critical reader's mother who began her nurse training in 1925. She demonstrates the kind of visionary professional care to which Heath refers, taking place almost 80 years ago:

> *After a short period of time, my mother became the sister of a long-stay ward for elderly women. There was only one other registered nurse and two enrolled nurses, the rest of the staff being completely untrained nursing auxiliaries and ward orderlies. Many patients had bedsores. Additionally, the ward stank of stale urine and most patients slept badly unless given sleeping pills. There was an air of hopelessness and apathy amongst patients and staff alike. Several patients had oral thrush. Anyone who thinks a professional problem-solving approach to nursing is relatively new is wrong. Faced with this horrifying scenario, the new sister called a ward staff meeting. She sympathised with the staff about the ancient equipment with which they tried to care for patients and said that she intended to go on the warpath on their patients' and their behalf. For their part, she trusted them to follow her lead in instituting nursing care to heal existing bedsores and prevent any more developing and to improve the lives of the patients.*
>
> *To this end she:*
> - *went to see the matron, who had been the matron of the original workhouse, and told her that the situation in the ward was disgraceful, that she intended to ensure that it was improved rapidly and that she knew the matron would give her every support;*
> - *collected 10 of the worst stained and smelling pillows, put them on a trolley and personally took them down to the sewing room, demanding their replacement with new pillows and washable, waterproof covers. She repeated this each week until all the pillows were unstained and sweet-smelling;*
> - *instituted two-hourly toileting for those who were incontinent, showing staff how to wash all wet areas of skin to remove urine;*

- used the now forgotten 'air rings' for patients to sit on, preventing sacral sores developing;
- showed staff how to lift and turn patients so that skin was not scraped across sheets in the process and so that, in each change of position, pressure was distributed to different areas;
- marched down to the kitchen and demanded a later supper hour after seeing that many patients appeared malnourished and identifying that they did not sleep because they were hungry, having had their last meal at 5 p.m. When told that there was no one in the kitchen to prepare a later supper, she had bread, butter and eggs sent up to the ward each day so that the ward orderly could prepare scrambled eggs and bread and butter as an evening snack, doing this herself on the first evening. She then asked the night staff to reduce the administration of sleeping pills until very few at all were given. Levels of daytime confusion in patients fell correspondingly, as did incontinence;
- worked with staff and observed them in all aspects of care. In this way she realised that the incidence of oral thrush was linked to the practice of one auxiliary of feeding a line of patients, each with his or her own bowl of pudding, using only one spoon which went from mouth to mouth. Some sessions on basic hygiene, always directed to obtaining co-operation and not alienating staff, were given, supported with encouragement of patients to feed themselves, whatever the resulting mess. The linen room was persuaded to supply large table napkins to replace the ancient bibs that were in use;
- cajoled anyone she thought could help into going into the ward for half-an-hour after evening visiting, given that some patients rarely had visitors, and putting on entertainments (this was in the days before the ubiquitous TV). I remember this particularly well, as I was dragooned into giving renditions on the ward piano, supported by a number of quavering sopranos, of gems such as 'Love's old sweet song'.

At the end of three months the smell of urine had gone, there were no bedsores and no oral thrush; the general appearance of the patients was far less skeletal and the outside world was, at least for some, remembered.

Fundamental values and principles

The way that nurses view older people strongly influences their work with them. Pursey and Luker (1995) highlight the distinction between nurses' attitudes to older people and the structural context of their work. They believe that, although some nurses may feel negative about working with older people, these negative views are not reflected in the care given. Instead attitudes are communicated in a variety of subtle ways.

Everyone has rights, irrespective of age. Civil rights should not be eroded or disregarded, which is often the case in certain environments for older people. The NHS and Community Care Act 1990 lists six core rights that should be maintained for everyone:

- The right of choice, with the opportunity to select independently from a range of options.
- The maintenance of all rights and entitlements associated with 'citizenship'.
- The potential for fulfilment through realization of personal aspirations and abilities in all aspects of daily life.
- The promotion of independence through the opportunity to think and act without reference to another person. This includes a willingness to incur a degree of calculated risk.
- The right to privacy.
- The right to dignity through the recognition of the intrinsic value of people by respecting their uniqueness and their personal need.

An older person may not be able to carry out all the activities required for daily independent life, but those that can be achieved should be maintained and those that cannot be mastered should be adapted. According to Drury (1996), care of the older person constitutes the best example of the absolute need for a seamless medical and social service. Each individual should be treated as a whole person with a variety of needs and guaranteed the same quality of service. Older people should be respected, have their confidentiality maintained, be involved in all decision making through appropriate and effective communication, and encouraged to be as independent as possible (Care Sector Consortium, 1998). Although these criteria were identified for the independent sector, they are applicable to all care environments.

According to Heath (1998), there is now overriding evidence that choice and control contribute to positive health outcomes and enhance both quality and quantity of life. Loss of control is associated with ill health, psychological distress and increased mortality. However, the ability to facilitate older people in promoting rights, responsibilities, choices and risk taking requires knowledge, understanding, sensitivity and skill. Ethical issues in nursing are linked to values and principles; they are considered in the next section.

ETHICAL AND LEGAL ISSUES RELATED TO WORKING WITH OLDER PERSONS

Ethical and legal issues

What attitudes do nurses have towards care of older people? What images do they have of their older patients? Does it matter, or can nurses overcome their own prejudices by 'being professional'? According to Masterson (1997), studies going back as far as the 1950s show that many nurses hold negative attitudes towards older people. She suggests that these attitudes may reflect the widespread negative stereotypes of old age in society generally. So how can looking at ethics help nurses as professionals? Ethics is the study of morals. Morality is concerned with good or bad in the human character and the distinction between right and wrong. Consideration of these may encourage you to look at how you arrive at some of the important decisions you are required to make in discharging your professional duties to your older patients.

Ethics tends to refer to customs, manners, sexuality, religious behaviour, and so on. It generally takes into account an individual's character and objective behaviour and the ideals that are being pursued. There are two principal approaches to ethics:

- **normative**: what people should do;
- **descriptive**: what people actually do.

Defining right and wrong

Theoretically, people should always do what is 'right', although in reality they may not. But how is 'right' defined? Is it in terms of consequences, 'the end justifies the means'? If so, is the end being sought for the good of an individual (ethical egoism), or the good of the greatest number of people (utilitarianism)? Or is 'right' defined in terms of the intrinsic value of the process, rather than the outcome? If so, people should do the right thing at any given moment in any given situation, regardless of the consequences.

Think about right and wrong, moral and amoral: where do they come from? Immanuel Kant (1724–1804) believed that all people are equal by the very nature of being human, regardless of who they are. So it would be wrong to behave differently towards some of your patients because, for example, they were older. This is known as the deontological approach to moral decision making, in which actions are regarded as intrinsically good or bad as determined by some higher standard.

In a teleological approach, an action is regarded as right in terms of the good produced as the consequence of an action. This approach was promoted by the group of philosophers known as the utilitarians, chiefly John Stuart Mill (1806–1873) and Jeremy Bentham (1748–1832). It was based on the 'greatest happiness principle': actions are right to the extent that they promote happiness, and wrong in proportion to the extent that they promote unhappiness (Mill, 1972).

These are personal-professional decisions and each situation is unique. It is impossible to give 'rules' for every eventuality in your day-to-day practice. It is more important that you have a chance to consider your approach in more depth than perhaps you have previously been able to. According to Ebersole and Hess (1998) and Heath (1998), ethics must be based on four principles essential to the care of older people:

- **principle of beneficence**: the assumption that, because of professional training, judgement and scientific inquiry, the professionals in organized institutions know what is in the best interests of the patient. The decisions must be made in an objective manner, so the results will produce greater good than harm.

- **principle of respect for autonomy**: the assumption that action which respects the values and the beliefs of the individual older patient is of utmost importance. Decisions are based on the preferences of the patient.
- **principle of justice**: the assumption that justice is achieved by the distribution of costs and benefits to the individual, the family and society.
- **principle of family responsibility**: the assumption that families are obliged to care for their own and that differences in understanding of these responsibilities can be negotiated.

The uncertainties surrounding ethical decisions are often what cause nurses the greatest concern, because there is no clear-cut guidance and they cannot draw on cut-and-dried rules or personal experiences. One can often deal with ethical issues more effectively if all the professional background information is available, since this reduces uncertainties. Here are some relevant questions:

- Are you clear about your legal position?
- Do you know the appropriate code of professional conduct for your work? An example is the NMC (2002) Code of Professional Conduct.
- Are you clear about the appropriate guidelines or codes of practice for your setting?
- Have you found out whether there are written or unwritten procedures (custom and practice) which apply?
- Are you aware of the preferences, practices and concerns of the older patients you are caring for?
- Do you know the health and safety laws that apply to your work area? Two examples are the Department of Health Health and Safety at Work Act 1974 and the Control of Substances Hazardous to Health (COSHH) Regulations.

If morals is about principles, then ethics is about practice. All nurses need to consider ethical issues because of the

- trust put in the nurse by the patient;
- patient's vulnerability;
- 'power' of the nurse;
- critical significance of the relationship (life or death).

Ethics enables us to decide which actions would be moral or immoral in a given situation. It provides the descriptive and analytical tools to ensure that we behave morally in our personal and professional lives. Professional ethics is not the same as personal morality. It consists of a set of rules specifically governing moral conduct in professionals.

Most of us, nurses included, come to decisions based on personal beliefs and value systems, yet 'the importance and influence of our personal beliefs, and their influence over our actions, is not always recognised. None the less ... values are the personal aspects and foundations of social and ethical living' (Tschudin, 1992). Our decisions can also be influenced by our perception of their potential effects on ourselves and others: What will happen if I do this? What will happen if I don't do this? What effect will that have on me? What effect will that have on others?

Ethics and older patients

According to Ebersole and Hess (1998), 'Medicine has had a long-standing ambition to forestall death, and because individuals more than 85 years old are the ones who most frequently die, the relentless drive to keep them alive has been evident. Less attention has been paid to the dignity of ageing and health'. Whether or not you agree with them, you will know that the ethical issues involved in caring for older patients are not straightforward. To Ebersole and Hess, these issues demand answers to questions like these:

- What is the nature of the nurse/patient relationship?
- Is the patient participating through choice and informed consent?
- What is the quality of life of the patient and the nurse?

Informed consent and advocacy

Ebersole and Hess feel that many older people grew up under the 'priestly model' of health and seem most comfortable with a 'whatever you say' approach to the health-care system. They argue that a belief in informed consent is basic to the relationship between patient and provider. Underlying such a belief are the ethical concepts of beneficence (charity and open-handedness) and respect for autonomy. The ethical principle of respect for autonomy is supported by the legal right to self-determination by any adult of sound mind. Professionals are obliged to obtain informed consent before proceeding with any therapeutic intervention.

Ebersole and Hess suggest three requirements for informed consent:

- adequate disclosure of information
- patient understanding of the information given
- a voluntary decision to undergo the procedure or intervention.

They suggest that nurses 'have an obligation to encourage and guide the client in seeking relevant information and to bolster the client's belief that he or she has a right to know'. To what extent should nurses act as advocates for their older patients? Suppose, for example, that you feel your patient cannot give informed consent and needs you to act or decide on their behalf.

Activity_____

- Although advocacy is an expectation set out in the Code of Professional Conduct, some organizations are not wholly in favour of advocacy. You may wish to bear this in mind and investigate the policies of the organizations with which you come into contact.

- Illness, lack of knowledge or inability to express themselves verbally can cause older patients to lose the power to represent themselves. At such times they may need someone else to act on their behalf or to become their advocate.
- Patients who are demented, deaf or have a learning disability may need an advocate. Who is best placed to play the advocacy role? Is it always the nurse? Do you think that an interpreter for patients whose mother tongue is not English, for example, could be an appropriate advocate?
- In the case study, Mary describes occasions when others acted as an advocate for her. See if you can identify where this happens and consider the effects on Mary.
- How could that advocacy have been handled differently, and with what result?

In paediatrics, nurses are likely to have developed a close relationship with the children in their care, and this means they are well placed to listen to the family, support the family and act as advocates for the child and their family. The same point could be made about nurses working with vulnerable older patients who also need listening to, support and perhaps advocacy.

Ebersole and Hess's advice on removing barriers to informed consent

- Whenever possible, remove the barriers to informed consent by reversing depression, controlling pain and reducing medications that impair decision making. In most cases this will successfully restore the patient's ability to participate fully in making decisions.
- When it is impossible to restore judgement and lucidity, decisions should be based on the patient's historic patterns. If the patient's preferences were discussed in the past, they should be respected. Ask questions such as these: What was important to the patient? What would the patient have decided based on those values? This guards against substitute judgements based on family desires. Nonetheless, you need to be aware that sometimes the patient's decision can have profound adverse effects on the family. When decisions are not clear-cut; an appropriate compromise may be required, if one can be found.
- Decisions should not be made by family members or the doctor based on their own values. Substitute judgement must be relied on when it is not possible to construct decisions based on knowledge of the older patient. In these cases beneficence is the main consideration. The person making the substitute judgement must be fully informed about the range of possibilities and their consequences.

- Notice the importance of being aware of your own values, so as to reduce the possibility of basing decisions on your values instead of the patient's values.

Ethics can be complex and challenging

The ethics of caring for older patients can be complex and challenging. Often there are no easy answers. Use the support of colleagues in your setting to discuss issues of ethics. Find out their values and clarify yours. Work to avoid imposing your values on your older patients.

LEGAL ISSUES

Your work is governed by the Code of Professional Conduct, the Scope of Professional Practice and the law. The legal information in this chapter may not be applicable to a specific case involving your practice. If you need help and advice, you should contact your union, the NMC or another professional body, and a solicitor. Most of the information here refers to the law in England and Wales. The legal situation in Scotland and Northern Ireland is likely to be different.

There is very little legislation in the UK relating to the performance of specific tasks by different types of health-care professional. Other countries give detailed instructions on who can do what. Here it is only some responsibilities that are specific; for example, a death certificate can normally be signed only by a doctor, although this is changing in some areas. Prescribing practice was the domain of doctors and sometimes dentists. This position changed in 2001 when legislation gave nurses and others the licence to prescribe (Department of Health, 2001).

The allocation of many individual tasks relating to professional practice has evolved as a result of custom and practice rather than as a legal directive. Sometimes this is appropriate, as it relates to the knowledge base and training provided to each profession. However, an objective examination of professional practice indicates that although there are core roles and tasks specific to a profession, an increasing number of areas are open to negotiation, certainly at the boundaries of professional practice.

'Reasonable' and 'reasonable care'

What if you were called to account for an action you had taken? The courts and/or the professional conduct mechanisms of the NMC would have to decide whether the action you had taken was 'reasonable'. The test of what is reasonable is based on the 1957 case of *Bolam v. Friern Barnet Hospital Management Committee*, which decided: 'The test is the standard of the ordinary skilled man exercising and professing to have that special skill. A man need not possess the highest expert skill at the risk of being found negligent: it is sufficient if he exercises the skill of an ordinary competent man exercising that particular art'.

Although this test originally applied to a doctor, the same test could be applied to a professional nurse whose actions have been called into question. In 1986 *Wilsher v. Essex Area Health Authority* set the standard of 'reasonable care' expected of students and junior staff. The standard is that of a reasonably competent practitioner and not that of a student or junior. In other words, the registered practitioner has a duty to ensure that any care delegated is carried out to a reasonably competent standard (Pyne, 1998).

Such rulings are helpful. You are not expected to be an expert, unless you profess to be. But you are expected to be a reasonably competent practitioner. You would be expected to know, and be able to articulate, the basis on which you had made any decision regarding care – evidence, research or experience, for example. You would need to be able to demonstrate that most reasonable practitioners would have acted in the same way as you did.

Experts and specialists

Who are experts and specialists? By the same argument as for 'reasonable care', if you professed to have knowledge and skills above that of the ordinary competent practitioner, then you would have to be able to justify that claim if you were called to account for actions taken as an expert or specialist. You can profess this extra knowledge explicitly (e.g. by virtue of your job title) or implicitly (by other means).

Duty of care

In law there exists a duty of care between nurses and their patients. The test of duty of care is the case of *Donoghue v. Stephenson* that arose when Mrs Donoghue drank a bottle of ginger beer manufactured by Stephenson that contained the remains of a dead snail, discovered when the bottle of ginger beer had been half-consumed. The Lord Atkin, judging the case, said: 'You must take reasonable care to avoid acts or omissions which you can reasonably foresee would be likely to injure your neighbour'. Who then in law is my neighbour? The answer seems to be 'persons who are so closely and directly affected by my act that I ought to have them in contemplation as being so affected when I am directing my mind to the acts or omissions that are called in question' (UKCC, 1996a).

It was found in the case of the bottle of ginger beer that the manufacturers owed a duty of care to the consumer. Nurses owe a duty of care to their patients, but not at all times and in all places. For a duty of care to exist there needs to be a pre-existing relationship. If, for example, a nurse is travelling to the shops and passes by an older person who has fallen, the nurse does not owe that person a duty of care as a nurse and is not legally required to stop and give assistance. You might, however, argue the morality of this situation. If the nurse did stop to offer help, then it would have been as a volunteer. If the nurse were employed to provide such assistance within a place of work, a duty of care would exist. However, if the nurse stops to give assistance, the injured older person is entitled to expect the same standard of care that would be provided by any other nurse in the same circumstances (Dimond, 1995).

In simple terms, a duty of care exists if the actions of one person can be seen as being reasonably foreseeable to affect or harm another. The Code of Professional Conduct (NMC, 2002) underlines this duty of care as revealed in the following statements:

- Act always in such a manner as to promote and safeguard the interests and well-being of patients.
- Ensure that no action or omission on your part, or within your sphere of responsibility, is detrimental to the interests, condition or safety of patients.

Consent

Adults have the right in law to choose whether to consent to their bodies being touched by another person. If this consent is not given, an offence of trespass to the person, or of battery (if actually touched), would be committed and the person touched would have the right to pursue an action through the civil courts (Dimond, 1995). The *Patient's Charter* (Department of Health, 1991) states that everyone is entitled 'to be given a clear explanation of any treatment proposed, including any risks and alternatives before they decide whether they agree to the treatment'. The mere giving of consent by a patient to a nurse or doctor is insufficient to prevent the person who gave that consent being able to pursue a legal action, although the patient would need to prove that the person who had obtained consent was in some way liable. For this reason, it is important that nurses consider carefully how consent is obtained before interventions and how they judge the competence of the older patient to give consent. This is particularly important as nursing practice is constantly changing and nurses are carrying out an increasing number of invasive procedures (Power, 1997).

When is consent valid?

Stauch (1998) states that for consent to be valid it must fulfil three criteria:

- The patient must be competent to give the consent.
- There must be no duress or undue influence upon the patient to give the consent.
- The patient must be suitably informed about the nature of the proposed intervention.

One test of competence for giving consent is known as Gillick competence. This requires that the person is able to understand, in broad terms, the nature and purpose of the proposed intervention. This has been further refined in another legal case where it was decided that the person must be able to take in and retain the information, believe the information and make a decision after balancing the facts (Stauch, 1998).

If some older patients are to be judged as competent, then others may be judged as not competent. Such patients might be those who are mentally ill or who are unconscious. Then no other person, except by a court order, can give consent on behalf of the patient, except a person with parental responsibility (Montgomery, 1998). Doctors can use their professional responsibility and privilege to decide that it is in the best interests of the patient to proceed with a treatment, and can do so even if the relatives disagree. This does not preclude discussion with relatives, nor does it mean that the relatives might not be asked to sign a consent form. Indeed the relatives might be asked to sign a consent form or enter into a discussion with the care team partly to make them included in the care and decision-making process. But then the consent would only indicate that a discussion had taken place; it would have no legal standing.

Forms of consent

Consent can be written, implied and word of mouth. Although consent in writing is common for surgical and invasive procedures, and also for procedures in which the degree of risk to the patient is greater than in less invasive procedures, the law does not require consent to be given in any particular way. However, it is clear that consent in writing is evidence which could be produced to defend a subsequent assault charge (Dimond, 1995). It is often believed that consent should be 'informed', but it is recognized that in the English legal system there is no requirement for the patient to be fully informed (Montgomery, 1998). The requirement is that the doctor should give the patient the information the doctor deems reasonable for the purpose of the patient deciding whether to accept or reject a proposed treatment. The appropriate precedents here are the Ms Sidaway case of 1985 and the Bolam test of 1957.

Amy Sidaway

Amy Sidaway suffered persistent neck and shoulder pain and was advised by her surgeon to have an operation on her spine to relieve it. Although she was told about the possibility of the operation disturbing a spinal root, she was not informed about the danger of damage to her spinal cord and the effects to her health should this happen. She gave consent and surgery was carried out. The operation left her with spinal cord damage and a serious level of disability. She sued the surgeon and the hospital, claiming that she had not been made aware of all the risks involved with the proposed surgery and that she was therefore not able to give informed consent. Ms Sidaway lost her appeal to the trial judge and later to the Court of Appeal.

She also appealed to the House of Lords. Lord Scarman, one of the lords who heard the case, said that, in his opinion, the surgeon was not in breach of his duty of care. Lord Bridge, another of the lords hearing the case, said that the information given to Ms Sidaway was appropriate and sufficient and that evidence had been obtained from other doctors about the operation and customs and practice in this field of surgery at that time (1985). He recounted that Ms Sidaway's one expert witness, another neurosurgeon, agreed readily and without reservation that the surgeon, now deceased, had followed a practice which would be accepted as proper by a responsible body of neurosurgeons. The Bolam test of professional negligence had been applied and the deceased surgeon was not found to be negligent or in breach of his duty of care (Hepple and Matthews, 1991). Amy Sidaway lost her appeal to the House of Lords.

Implied consent

Implied consent is the consent implied by the non-verbal responses of the patient. Examples of implied consent include an older patient who opens her mouth for a thermometer to be put in it, and an older person who rolls up a sleeve so that blood pressure can be taken as the nurse approaches with a sphygmomanometer. However, this can be dangerous as the nurse may take the blood pressure first and then give an injection immediately following. The patient has not necessarily intended to imply consent for the latter, despite the fact that he has diabetes and has often had injections. For this reason, spoken consent is preferable.

Word-of-mouth consent

Word-of-mouth or spoken consent occurs when the patient agrees verbally to a treatment or intervention being carried out. It does not necessarily mean that the patient understands the reasons for the treatment or intervention. Care should be exercised that the test of competence mentioned by Stauch (1998) is applied before seeking consent. This is particularly important when dealing with a confused older person. The NMC affirms that you must obtain consent before you can give any treatment or care.

Informed consent

It would appear that, in the eyes of the law, no one else can give consent on behalf of the older patient. But could we argue that the test of competence should be satisfied before any other action is taken to force the patient to be treated? Provided that at the time the consent was given the person was judged as competent to give it, then the fact that they subsequently become mentally impaired or less competent does not invalidate the consent (Dimond, 1995). If there is doubt about the competence of the older patient, the doctor can proceed anyway, using their privilege and professional responsibility to do what is believed to be in the best interests of the patient. Informed consent is a process, not a single moment in time. Information often has to be given to patients over time if it cannot be absorbed all at once. Sometimes it takes time to build trust. Ask yourself how urgently the consent is required. And remember, consent is a two-way process. The doctor or nurse has to learn enough about the patient to make a decision as well. Furthermore, in hospitals you may need to view proxy consent in the light of hospital organization.

Negligence

In law, for negligence to be judged to have occurred, it must be established that

- a duty of care existed;
- there has been a breach of that duty;
- a breach of the duty of care was reasonably foreseeable.

In these situations the Bolam test is usually applied. So would another nurse of a similar standing, education and experience have foreseen that the event might have occurred? If yes, negligence might have occurred and the nurse might be judged as negligent. The other component to be established is causation. Can it be proved that the event being cited as due to negligence by the nurse was actually caused by the nurse, or might it have been due to something or someone else?

Negligence and the importance of record-keeping

Careful and accurate record-keeping may assist the nurse in defending claims of negligence. Reasons for decisions need to be recorded, as well as the actual interventions undertaken. The NMC continues to hold that records should 'identify problems that have arisen and the action taken to rectify them and provide evidence of the care planned, the decisions made, the care delivered and the information shared' (UKCC, 1998). The NMC also believes that your records should demonstrate 'evidence that you have understood and honoured your duty of care, that you have taken all reasonable steps to care for the patient and that any actions or omissions on your part have not compromised their safety in any way' (UKCC, 1998).

Emphasizing the legal aspects of accountability

Following the report *Not Because They Are Old* (Health Advisory Service 2000, 1998), the government announced that standards of care for older patients who are cared for by the NHS are to be developed and implemented. The government recognized that 'staff and patients have different understandings about their care, often because there has not been a clear explanation about what is happening, and why. Staff do not always effectively negotiate the "boundaries of care" with patients and relatives' (Health Advisory Service 2000, 1998). The new standards will attempt to require providers of care for older patients to account for what is delivered.

Activity

Learn about the *Graham Pink* case (Pink, 1994). Graham Pink was a night charge nurse at Stepping Hill Hospital. Between 1989 and 1990 he became concerned about standards of care and took his concerns to the newspapers. He eventually lost his job because, his employers argued, he had breached patient confidentiality in the information he had given the papers. If you would like to find out what happened to Mr Pink, you could carry out a literature search of the *Nursing Times* and the *Guardian*, and contact the BBC about the documentary it made.

Nurses are professionally accountable for their actions. The Code of Professional Conduct (NMC, 2002) is clear that no one else can answer for you and you cannot sidestep your responsibility by saying that you were acting on someone else's orders. You are accountable to yourself, too. Keeping a reflective diary is one way of accounting for your thoughts and actions. It also provides you with a way of learning from situations and of discussing points later with your clinical supervisor (Johns and Freshwater, 1998), mentor or preceptor, practice supervisor or assessor.

No one person, rule, code of practice or guideline can tell you what to do in every situation. But the Code of Professional Conduct (NMC, 2002) sets out the following important principles:

- Maintain and improve professional knowledge and competence.
- Acknowledge limitations in knowledge and competence.
- Decline any duty or responsibility unless you are able to perform it in a safe and skilled manner.

Confidentiality

Nurses are required to protect all confidential information concerning patients and clients obtained in the course of professional practice and to make disclosures only with consent, where required by the order of a court, or where disclosure can be justified in the wider public interest (NMC, 2002). Dimond (1995) lists exceptions to the duty of confidentiality:

- consent of a patient
- interests of a patient
- court orders
- subpoena
- Supreme Court Act 1981
- statutory duty to disclose
- Road Traffic Act 1972
- Prevention of Terrorism Act 1989
- Public Health Act 1984
- Misuse of Drugs Act 1971
- public interest
- police.

Nurses are required to protect patient confidentiality by the terms of their employment contracts (usually) and through their duty of care. To trust someone else with private and personal information is a very important matter, so make sure they preserve the spirit of trust in which it was given.

What must be kept confidential?

Sometimes it can be difficult to determine what information should be confidential. Are patients' middle names or their postcodes confidential? Both are publicly accessible, easily gleaned from electoral registers in public libraries. However, in the nursing situation, the information has been given freely to nurses in the performance of his or her professional role and should be treated as confidential. The easiest way to manage the dilemma of what is and isn't confidential is to treat all information as confidential. Check with the older patient in your care about the more obvious information you might be asked to divulge; for example, is the patient happy for you to divulge their religious beliefs to the visiting minister of religion?

A further dilemma occurs when the older patient has been discovered to be suffering from a terminal illness or disease. Questions arise such as: Should the patient be told? Or should the relatives be told first and then asked for their opinion as to what is disclosed to the patient? This is not an uncommon situation. Nurses, doctors, relatives and almost everyone else close to the patient knows the person's diagnosis and prognosis. The patient may be kept in the dark by professionals and family who judge that non-disclosure will protect this person. What of patients' rights to confidentiality, autonomy and respect? Once the option to tell the relatives is enacted, a conspiracy of silence can begin (Dimond, 1995).

In law, patients have a right to information about their state of health and also for this information to be kept confidential. This means that to tell the relatives would indeed breach the patient's right to confidentiality, and could thus become the subject of a complaint, either through local processes or by recourse to the courts. It is for the patient to decide if and when the family is told. This position should be upheld and respected. There are occasions when the patient is too ill to be informed, hence they can no longer make independent decisions. In this case, a relative's viewpoint on care and treatment might be required. However, these occasions should be the exception not the rule.

SUMMARY

This chapter looked at the dimensions of professional practice. It considered the notion of professional practice and the characteristics relating to a professional entity. It charted the course of becoming a professional nurse through the process of education, training and embracing the norms of professional practice through regulatory practice. The Code of Professional Conduct was described from different health and social care disciplines, illustrating the similarities and differences between them. The notion of accountability was elaborated with emphasis on what it means to be an autonomous practitioner. Ethical and legal issues are central to all professional practice. They were discussed with particular relevance to older people. Finally, there is a duty to give care of a professional standard. Failure to provide care of the right standard is considered to be negligent. Negligence is clearly a breach of professional practice and this chapter examined a nurse's duty of care. For the most part, nurses and health professionals keep within the guidelines and demands inherent within codes of professional conduct.

Caring for older people is a challenging task and constantly makes moral and ethical demands on health-care practitioners. It is a health-care practitioner's duty to ensure that they and others do not abuse their position when caring for vulnerable old people. Caring for older people is a unique privilege that can be most enjoyable, full of humour, care and compassion. And nursing older people can enable all nurses and health-care professionals to develop personally and professionally in areas that underpin all health and social care. Instead of being the Cinderella that is often portrayed, it should have central importance in our caring services. Consequently, raising the profile of elder care is the duty of all concerned with health and social care.

◀ **Key points**

1 Professional legal duty with respect to accountability and responsibility.
2 Description of a profession.
3 Requirements for professional nursing practice.
4 Management of registration.
5 Codes of professional conduct and concepts identified therein.
6 Explanations of care, caring, cure and health.
7 Continuing professional development and the need for lifelong learning.
8 The importance of clinical governance, research and audit.
9 Working with older people.
10 How to use the empowerment model in elderly care situations.
11 Partnership working.
12 Fundamental values and principles.
13 Ethical and legal issues.

REFERENCES

Audit Commission (1995) *United They Stand*. Audit Commission, London.
Audit Commission (1997) *The Coming of Age: Improving Care Services for Older People*. Audit Commission, London.
Basford, L. (2003) The context of care. In: *Theory and Prctice of Nursing: An Integrated Approach to Caring Practice* (ed. Basford, L and Slevin, O.). Nelson Thornes, Cheltenham, Glos., pp. 42–72.
Blytheway, B. (1995) *Rethinking Ageing: Ageism*. Open University Press, Buckingham.
Care Sector Consortium (1998) *The New Care Awards*. Healthwork, London.
Clarke, A. (1991) Nurses as role models and health educators. *Journal of Advanced Nursing*, **16**, 1178–1184.
Davies, C. A. (1996a) Cloaked in a tattered illusion. *Nursing Times*, **92**(45), 44–46.

Davies, C. A. (1996b) New vision of professionalism. *Nursing Times*, **92**(46), 54–56.

Department of Health (1974) *Health and Safety at Work Act*. The Stationery Office, London.

Department of Health (1990) *NHS and Community Care Act*. The Stationery Office, London.

Department of Health (1991) *The Patient's Charter*. The Stationery Office, London.

Department of Health (1999) *Better Care, Higher Standards: A Charter for Long-Term Care*. The Stationery Office, London.

Department of Health (2001) *National Service Framework for Older People*. The Stationery Office, London.

Dimond, B. (1995) *Legal Aspects of Nursing*, 2nd edn. Prentice Hall, London.

Drury, M. (1996) Introduction. In: *A Guide to Care of the Elderly* (ed. Shukla, R. B. and Brooks, D.). The Stationery Office, London.

Ebersole, P. and Hess, P. (1998) *Towards Healthy Ageing: Human Needs and Nursing Response*, 5th edn. Mosby, Princeton NJ.

Elston, M. (1991) The politics of professional power: medicine in a changing health service. In: *The Sociology of the Health Service* (ed. Gabe, J., Calnar, M. and Bury, M.). Routledge, London.

Health Advisory Service 2000 (1998) *Not Because They Are Old: An Independent Inquiry into the Care of Older People on Acute Wards in General Hospitals*. Health Advisory Service 2000, London.

Heath, H. (1998) Care of the older person. In: *Nursing Practice and Health Care: A Foundation Text*, 3rd edn (ed. Hinchliff, S., Norman, S. and Schober, J.). Arnold, London.

Hepple, B. A. and Matthews, M. H. (1991) *Tort: Cases and Materials*, 4th edn. Butterworth, London.

Johns, C. (1996) The benefits of a reflective model of nursing. *Nursing Times*, **92**(27), 3941.

Johns, C. and Freshwater, D. (1998) *Transforming Nursing through Reflective Practice*. Blackwell Science, Oxford.

Lancely, A. (1985) Use of controlling language in rehabilitation of the elderly. *Journal of Advanced Nursing*, **10**(2), 125–135.

Littler, G. (1997) Social age-cohort control: a theory. *Journal of the British Society of Gerontology*, **7**(3), 11–13.

Macmillan Open Learning (1997) *Influences in Health Care: Media Perspectives*. Macmillan Magazines, London.

Masterson, A. (1997) *The Continuing Care of Older People*, UKCC Policy Paper 1. UKCC, London.

Mill, J. S. (1972) *Utilitarianism* (ed. Warnock, M.). Fontana, London.

Montgomery, J. (1998) *Health Care Law*. Oxford University Press, Oxford.

Nazarko, L. (1998) Continuity of care for older people. *Nursing Standard*, **12**(52) 42–45.

Newton, E. (1980) *This Bed My Centre*. Virago, London.

NMC (2001) *Nursing and Midwifery Order*. Queen's Printer, London.

NMC (2002) *Code of Professional Conduct*. Nursing and Midwifery Council, London.

NMC (2003) *Professional Conduct Annual Report (2002–2003)*. Nursing and Midwifery Council, London.

Pennels, C. (1997) Nursing and the law: clinical responsibility. *Professional Nurse*, **13**(3), 162–164.

Pink, G. (1994) The price of truth: ethics at the bedside. *British Medical Journal*, **309**, 1700–1705.

Porter, S. (1990) Vain aspirations. *Nursing Times*, **86**(11), 46–47.

Power, K. (1997) The legal and ethical implications of consent to nursing procedures. *British Journal of Nursing*, **6**(15), 885–888.

Pursey, A. and Luker, K. (1995) Attitudes and stereotypes: nurses' work with older people. *Journal of Advanced Nursing*, **22**, 547–555.

Pyne, R. (1998) *Professional Discipline in Nursing, Midwifery and Health Visiting*, 3rd edn. Blackwell, Oxford.

Redfern, S. J. (1991) The elderly person: the challenge of an aged society. In: *Nursing Elderly People*, 2nd edn (ed. Redfern, S. J.). Churchill Livingstone, Edinburgh.

Rogers, C. (1961) *On Becoming a Person*. Houghton Mifflin, Boston MA.

Schön, D. A. (1992) The crisis of professional knowledge and the pursuit of the epistemology of practice. *Journal of Interprofessional Care*, **6**(1), 49–63.

Slevin, O. (2003) A nursing perspective of older people: the problem of ageism. In: *Theory and Practice of Nursing: An Integrated Approach to Patient Care*, 3rd edn (ed. Basford, L. and Slevin, O.). Nelson Thornes, Cheltenham, Glos., pp. 97–111.

Stauch, M. (1998) Consent in medical law. *British Journal of Nursing*, 7(2), 84.

Tones, B. and Tilford, S. (1994) *Health Education: Effectiveness, Efficiency and Equity*, 2nd edn. Chapman Hall, London.

Tschudin, V. (1992) *Ethics in Nursing*. Butterworth-Heinemann, Oxford.

UKCC (1986) *Project 2000: A New Preparation for Practice*. United Kingdom Central Council, London.

UKCC (1992a) *Code of Professional Conduct for the Nurse, Midwife and Health Visitor*, 3rd edn. United Kingdom Central Council, London.

UKCC (1992b) *Scope of Professional Practice*. United Kingdom Central Council, London.

UKCC (1995) *Standards for Post-registration Education and Practice (PREP)*. United Kingdom Central Council, London.

UKCC (1996a) *Guidelines for Professional Practice*. United Kingdom Central Council, London.

UKCC (1996b) *Position Statement on Clinical Supervision*. United Kingdom Central Council, London.

UKCC (1997) *The Nursing and Health Visiting Contribution to the Continuing Care of Older People*. United Kingdom Central Council, London.

UKCC (1998) *Guidelines for records and record keeping*. United Kingdom Central Council, London.

UKCC (2002) *Code of Professional Conduct*, 2nd edn. United Kingdom Central Council, London.

Victor, C. R. (1999) What is old age? In: *Nursing Older People*, 3rd edn (ed. Redfern, S. J. and Ross, F. M). Churchill Livingstone, Edinburgh.

Vollmer, H. M. and Mills, D. L. (1996) *Professionalisation*. Prentice-Hall, Englewood Cliffs, NJ.

Vousden, M. (1998) The highway code. *Nursing Times*, **94**(47), 31.

Wade, L. (1996) The social world of older people. In: *A Textbook of Gerontological Nursing: Perspectives on Practice* (ed. Wade, L. and Waters, S. K.). Baillière Tindall, London.

Wade, L. and Waters, S. K. (eds) (1995) *A Textbook of Gerontological Nursing: Perspectives on Practice*. Baillière Tindall, London.

WHO (1978) *Primary Health Care: A Report on the Conference on Primary Care*. World Health Organization, Geneva.

WHO (1984) *Health Promotion: A WHO Discussion Document on the Concepts and Principles*. WHO Regional Office for Europe, Copenhagen.

LEGAL CASES

Bolam v. Friern Barnet Hospital Management Committee (1957) All ER 118

Wilsher v. Essex Area Health Authority (1986) 3 All ER 801 [1987] 1 QB 730 [1987] 2 WLR 425

Sidaway v. Bethlem Royal Hospital Governors and Others (1985) 1 All ER 643

5 Developing Evidence-Based Practice

OBJECTIVES

- Describe what is meant by a best-practice model.
- Define evidence-based practice.
- Describe the major barriers and benefits to using sound evidence to support your practice with older people.
- Discuss the importance of using contemporary evidence in your own practice.
- Describe the research process.
- Describe the process of conducting a thorough literature review on any topic.
- Conduct a literature review on a topic of choice and demonstrate the strategy that you implemented to record essential data relevant to your selected documents.
- Identify and obtain information from key websites.
- Describe the essential components in conducting a critical appraisal of any research article or report.
- Identify several basic statistics that are reported in research reports and articles.
- Identify and define key concepts central to research.

INTRODUCTION

This chapter is an overview of evidence-based practice (E-BP) and the research process, two essential aspects of being an informed health-care professional. It is vital that you keep abreast of innovations from the Department of Health, partly because these changes directly affect your practice. This book contains many references to Department of Health documents on older people. If you have a good understanding of evidence and sources of evidence, then you can use this to inform your practice.

Research is proposed as the major source of evidence, so this chapter gives an overview of the research process, but many textbooks give a more in-depth study of the research process. At this stage, there are two important skills for you to master: conducting a thorough literature review and critically analysing the reports you obtain. These skills are described here in some detail. Try to apply these skills as you read the book as they do take time to develop.

EVOLUTION OF EVIDENCE-BASED PRACTICE

In 1978 the World Health Organization (WHO) and the United Nations Children's Fund (UNICEF) sponsored an international conference that met in Alma Ata, in Kazakhstan. This conference provided a significant declaration that supports basic health for all people conceptualized as primary health care. Central to this model of providing health care is the need to employ scientifically sound evidence as a basis for practice. Importantly, this requirement persists at all levels of health-care practice: international, national, local and individual. Thus, health-care practitioners (physicians, nurses, pharmacists, therapists, etc.) are obliged to know and to implement current E-BP in their respective fields. The implication of this declaration is that all health-care professionals need to be taught skills essential to critical appraisal.

Also in the 1970s, Archie Cochrane (1972) published his seminal book *Effectiveness and Efficiency: Random Reflections on Health Services*. Two decades later, he founded the Cochrane Collaboration with representatives from nine countries. Cochrane's ideas resulted in the creation of databases that house systematic reviews on research and practice. The goals of its centres around the world are to address three major aims of E-BP:

- **effectiveness**: basing health-care interventions on evidence-based empirical interventions.
- **efficiency**: essentially addressing cost-effectiveness in use of resources.
- **equality**: relating primarily to access to health care and the allocation of resources.

The initial focus of the Cochrane Collaboration centres was on documenting evidence based on quantitative research methods using the randomized controlled trial (RCT) as the gold standard. In 1998 the Cochrane Qualitative Methods Network expanded its mandate to include qualitative research in its review process (Qualitative Methods Network, 1999).

In response to this initiative, the medical profession revised the teaching and practice of medicine, promoting evidence-based medicine (E-BM). Sackett *et al.* (1996) define EB-M as 'the conscientious, explicit, and judicious use of current best evidence in making decisions about the care of individual patients' (p. 71). This definition point to the significance of both physician and patient making a knowledgeable choice, specific decisions being made and implemented, and the need for evaluating the outcomes of this decision. Estabrooks (1998, p. 18) outlines various criticisms lodged against the E-BM movement:

Some of the criticisms may be valid, others reactionary. Criticism in itself is healthy for any new intellectual undertaking. However, it is safe to say that EBM is more than a way of practising; it has taken on the qualities of a social movement whose purpose is, in part, and in addition to the obvious, the redistribution of power in medicine. If the movement is successful, the power base will move from the clinical

> *specialists and sub-specialists to the clinical epidemiologists who are both the producers and the purveyors of the new knowledge needed for EBM.*

Although a relative newcomer to this movement of using evidence to guide practice, nurse leaders contemplated how to use nursing research findings since the 1970s (Estabrooks, 1998). In the UK, Briggs (1972) documents the need for research as a basis for practice within the profession of nursing. Recently, Stone *et al.* (2002) report, 'Basing nursing practice on the best available evidence is now the expected standard of care' (p. 277). Mulhall (1998) defines evidence-based nursing (E-BN) as 'care concerning the incorporation of evidence from research, clinical expertise, and patient preferences into decisions about the health care of individual patients' (p. 5). It is notable that Kitson (2002) observes that the construct of E-BN is frequently used in nursing settings today, despite the 'many tensions in the way it was being interpreted, promoted and applied' (p. 179). Kitson also speculates about the future use of E-BN or E-BP when she comments:

> *The tension between the EBP movement and the patient-centred health-care movement embodies the philosophical and ideological tension between health-care as objective scientific endeavour and health-care as encounters with individuals bounded in unique time and context, requiring both the objective analysis of the scientist and the humanitarian connectedness of the healer-practitioner. (ibid., p. 181)*

Estabrooks (1998) and Kitson (2002), among others, argue for a broader interpretation of what constitutes evidence for purposes of practice knowledge in nursing. A common assumption is that the 'evidence in evidence-based practice is scientific fact derived from scientifically sound individual studies' (Estabrooks, 1998, p. 27). Rather than simply accepting the RCT as the *sine qua non* and the only source of evidence, Kitson concludes:

> *Definitions of evidence need to be understood in the context of establishing effective therapeutic relationships with clients and by balancing evidence from patients, clinical experience and research in order to arrive at the best clinical decision for care. ... [But,] as a discipline, it still needs to do a lot more describing, refining and classifying of basic constructs and concepts before it can put great reliance on the evidence that emerges from intervention studies alone. (ibid., p. 185)*

Similarly, Estabrooks (1998) acknowledges the need to contemplate non-research evidence (e.g. clinical experience and clinical judgement) and notes that this evidence is the most difficult of all to assess. This debate about what constitutes evidence continues in the literature. French (2002) provides an enlightening discussion on the concept of E-BN. There is an assumption that the term has meaning and many professionals adopt the goal of E-BN, and generally E-BP, as a *fait accompli*.

Pearson (2003) suggests 'evidence-based practice is the combination of individual clinical and professional expertise with the best available external evidence to produce practice that is most likely to lead to a positive outcome for a client or patient' (p. 321). However, French (2002) proposes that 'E-BP is in fact a product of the conceptual overlapping of already existing traditions' (p. 255). These overlapping practices, all of which are integral to health-care professions, include research-based practice, information management process, professional practice development, clinical judgement/problem solving, and managed care (French, 2002). He concludes, 'It is difficult to find any empirical evidence (research) to support the notion that the term "evidence" is a stable construct or that EBP is a distinct process which offers more than a novelty effect in a basically political scenario' (French, 2002, p. 255).

Kitson *et al.* (1998) extend this discussion on the concept of evidence when they describe the relationships between the nature of the evidence, context and facilitation as influential factors affecting the successful implementation of evidence in practice. For example, they propose that context entails organizational culture, leadership and measurement, concluding that 'the term itself does little to reflect the complexity of the concept' (McCormack *et al.*, 2002, p. 94). Other elements of the context to be taken into account include 'systems of decision-making, staff relationships, organizational systems, power differentials and the potential of the organization to innovate' (McCormack *et al.*, 2002, p. 101). These authors contend that implementing evidence into practice is compromised to the extent that the concept of context remains unclear. In a similar vein, Kitson and her colleagues confirm that the concept of facilitation is a complex one that requires further research to clarify the roles and relationships among various factors (Kitson *et al.*, 1998).

In the UK, 'clinical supervision provides a framework for self-regulation and developing informed deliberative practice, emphasizing not only self-monitoring through reflection on action, but also encouraging reflection in action' (Freshwater, 2003, p. 113). Although this framework is best developed in mental health, midwifery and child protection work, it is a relatively new development in other facets of nursing. Clinical supervision aims to support nurses to further develop their knowledge and skills for enhancing their practice. Furthermore, clinical supervision aims to bring practitioners and skilled supervisors together to reflect on practice, to identify solutions to problems, to increase understanding of professional issues, and importantly, to improve standards of care. Clinical supervision and E-BP share a common goal – providing the best possible care to all patients.

It is clear that the E-BP movement is established and moving forward. The literature is replete with different perspectives that either support or refute the validity of adopting a best-practice approach to providing care. To further the debate, Jennings and Loan (2001) recommend an international conference 'to consider the conflicting and controversial aspects of EBP' (p. 126). These comments highlight the need to develop a capacity for critical thinking and critical appraisal of evidence before applying ideas to practice. E-BP allows you to

- inform or advise patients accurately;
- make better use of limited resources;
- make appropriate and up-to-date interventions;
- measure practice against appropriate guidelines or standards.

Here are two websites featuring the development of E-BP skills:

- Oxford Workshops on Teaching Evidence-Based Medicine (http://cebm.jr2.ox.ac.uk/docs)
- workshopsteaching.html
- Oxford Workshops on How to Practise Evidence-Based Medicine (http://cebm.jr2.ox.ac.uk/docs/workshopsdoing.html)

Activity

- Define best practice in your own words. Identify three implications for best practice when providing care to your older patients.
- Select two references from the literature and identify three key differences between E-BM and E-BN.
- How would you explain the tension that Kitson (2002) identifies between E-BP and patient-centred health care?

MARY'S COMMENTS

Mary's comments about the broken leg

I don't know, but I broke that leg. I'd only stepped across the road and fell over. I tripped and went flying. The physio came here; she came here twice a week to give me exercises when I got out of the plaster. I was in plaster for three months and she thought I'd torn my tendon at the back.

Mary's comments about the broken hip

Whether I've damaged it again, I don't know. I think I may have done when I fell. I was at the top of the stairs and I turned to come down: I was more or less coming down backwards and I missed my footing.

I still try to do the exercises they tell me to do with the hip; it is very difficult and it does hurt sometimes. I do try; admittedly I don't do them as often as I should. She said I should do it ten times. I can't always do it so I do two or three when I first stand up, perhaps on the crutches, you know, after I want to get up to go to the toilet or something, but I don't do ten all at once – I just can't. I do try and do some at least during the day; it is only a couple of small exercises, one sort of lifting the leg and then another one. She said it was like ballet dancing. There were two of us and she said: 'You can do them together.'

Activity

- What evidence do you have from Mary about her situation?
- Identify other sources of evidence that can help you to clarify Mary's situation.
- What conclusions do you infer from Mary's comments?

KEY BARRIERS AND BENEFITS OF USING E-BP

Pearson (2003) comments, 'Most health professions are increasingly embracing the use of evidence-based guidelines to inform (rather than direct) practice and this is in response to high profile initiatives of governments and provider agencies' (p. 320). In the UK, the National Institutes of Health are poised to produce clinical guidelines based on reviews of research and the conduct of meta-analyses. This mandate to discover the best evidence available is intended to arm all health-care practitioners with the knowledge to excel in their practice. Thus, the literature is mounting as professionals, researchers and practitioners describe their findings and experiences (e.g. Angel *et al.*, 2000; Retsas, 2000). In one study, Angel *et al.* report the findings from a longitudinal quasi-experimental design to assess changes in knowledge and critical-thinking performance among nursing students ($n = 142$). Angel *et al.* note significant changes in knowledge acquisition as well as the quality and quantity of critical-thinking behaviours. Their findings lead them to conclude that faculty members need to employ evidence-based models to support decisions on teaching methodologies.

Cooper *et al.* (2001) explore 'the feasibility of introducing interdisciplinary education within undergraduate health professional programmes' (p. 228). From their systematic review, 141 studies emerge, 30 (21%) of which were included in the analysis. Of the 30 studies, 16 are evaluation studies and 14 are research studies. They conclude, 'Student health professionals were found to benefit from interdisciplinary education with outcome effects primarily relating to changes in knowledge, skills, attitudes and beliefs' (Cooper *et al.*, 2001, p. 228).

Retsas (2000) describes the use of research evidence by nurses working in a medical centre. Of the full-time staff nurses, 400 (50% response rate) returned the questionnaire, which was on barriers to research utilization. Retsas observes that 'staff at the medical centre have a high level of research readiness and share a strong sense of valuing the contribution that research can make to improving their practice' *(ibid.,* p. 605). Nonetheless, these staff members identify time as the major barrier to research utilization. Thus, Retsas recommends that organizational administrators ensure time to consider new ideas and read research reports and that appropriate facilities are provided to achieve these goals.

Whereas these authors document the use of E-BP in their research, other writers note several barriers to using E-BP. For instance, Pearson (2003, pp. 323–324) lists five criticisms that hinder the use of E-BP:

- Nurses are already doing it.
- Evidence-based nursing is 'cookbook' care.
- E-BP relies on randomized clinical trials and meta-analyses.
- There is no evidence.
- Theory is more important than evidence in guiding practice.

The first barrier is acceptable if one acknowledges that much of nursing practice is based on research findings. Nevertheless, directly related to implementing E-BP are the many barriers associated with the lack of skills to understand research reports, lack of critical skills to analyse research, time constraints, limited access to literature, and organizational constraints (DiCenso and Cullum, 1998). The second barrier implies that health-care professionals automatically follow guidelines without considering the individual's unique presentation. DiCenso and Cullum suggest that patient preferences and clinical expertise may override research evidence. To date, the RCT is deemed to be the gold standard. However, there is considerable activity in developing new protocols to include other research methods.

Pearson notes that RCTs may be the best source of evidence on effectiveness, and DiCenso and Cullum note that nurses often use qualitative approaches to assess patients' experiences, attitudes and beliefs. Although work is under way to establish protocols for systematic reviews of qualitative research, the lack of tools currently hinders widespread use of these research findings. Proponents of qualitative research methods assert that they are rigorous, albeit not in the same way as quantitative research methods. The fourth barrier recognizes that there is a dearth of nursing research to address nursing questions (Pearson, 2003). This finding is not surprising, given the relatively short history of nursing research activity (Hunt, 2001). Pearson argues that theory may be the focus of practice partly because evidence is often short-lived.

Activity

- Identify the major difference among the studies by Angel *et al.* (2000), Cooper *et al.* (2001) and Retsas (2000).
- Describe in your own words what you deem to be the major barrier to you implementing evidence in your practice with older people.
- Describe one barrier and one benefit to implementing E-BP in Mary's situation, based on Mary's comments (p. 12).

A LEARNING ENVIRONMENT THAT SUPPORTS KNOWLEDGE SHARING

Learning environments are typically classrooms, libraries and homes. Over the past decades, changes within work settings, such as loss of jobs, career changes, de-skilling and multi-skilling demands, and casualization of employment contracts, require educators and employers to rethink on-the-job training. Davies (2003) recognizes that

> *the meaning of work is shifting under these new circumstances, which demand learning renewal throughout a working life. ... Work is increasingly the site where pre-formulated and 'textbook' knowledge is being transformed into new knowledge and where new paradigms for knowing and learning are emerging. (p. 126)*

In his seminal book *The Fifth Discipline: The Art and Practice of the Learning Organization*, Senge (1990) introduces the concept of learning organizations. In creating this learning environment, Senge (1996) suggests that individuals at all levels of the organization take on a leadership role. For instance, he explains that these individuals are the '"seed carriers" of the new culture, who can move freely about the organization to find those who are predisposed to bringing about change, help out in organizational experiments, and aid in the diffusion of new learnings' (p. 46). If organizational administrators fail to espouse values and beliefs integral to promoting a learning culture, Kitson (2002) cautions that positive change regarding the development and use of E-BP will be hampered. Health-care administrators need to establish learning environments to support their staff members by providing access to technology and time to obtain critical evidence. Furthermore, commitment to this significant goal is demonstrated when administrators provide opportunities for staff development. In turn, organizational members need to embrace the concept of lifelong learning and accept their responsibility in remaining open and receptive to all learning experiences.

Caramanica *et al.* (2002) describe 'a collaboration between healthcare and academic organizations that supports evidence-based nursing practice' (p. 27). The goal of this collaboration is to support professional nurses and nursing students in basing their practice decisions on the best available evidence. Among the strategies employed, the authors describe research round-tables, conferences, author talks and use of a website. Maljanian *et al.* (2002) explain the research round-tables. Through a series of interactive and informal meetings, novice nurse researchers and nursing students are guided to learn 'the skill sets required to apply evidence base into nursing practice and to conduct outcome studies to derive new evidence' (Maljanian *et al.*, 2002, p. 86). In the four main sessions, topics include searching the literature, two sessions on critiquing the literature, and E-BP and outcomes research.

Maljanian *et al.* recommend the replication of research round-tables in other settings, along with other strategies, to advance the goal of providing E-BP in nursing.

This discussion supports the necessity of lifelong learning and places some responsibility on organizational administrators. These administrators need to be proactive in identifying and addressing their own organizational learning needs and in supporting their staff development.

Activity

- Identify the characteristics of the setting in which you learn best.
- Describe how your colleagues and tutor support your learning needs.
- Identify a topic you would like to pursue for improving the care of older people.
- For the topic you have just identified, write three key questions you could answer by doing a literature review.

The gold standard is evidence based on research. Research is comprehensively reviewed in many texts (e.g. Burns and Grove, 2001; Polit and Hungler, 1999) and will not be considered here. But to help you understand the linkages between research and evidence, here is an overview of the research process.

COMPONENTS OF THE RESEARCH PROCESS

Burns and Grove (2001) define research as 'diligent and systematic inquiry or investigation to validate and refine existing knowledge and generate new knowledge' (p. 3). Research is a process that entails several components:

- background information on the concept of interest, topic or problem
- literature review (see p. 118)
- problem and purpose statements
- methodology
- design, including ethical considerations
- sample and population
- methods of measurement
- data collection and analysis
- results or findings
- interpretation and conclusions
- dissemination of findings.

All research begins with a hunch or idea about some phenomenon. Hence, because it is rare to identify a phenomenon that has not been investigated previously, there is typically background information that can set the stage for the research. For instance, it is possible to identify the historical development of a concept and various, sometimes conflicting, definitions. An in-depth literature review is essential to discover what research has been conducted on that phenomenon, the key findings, the methods used, and the conclusions drawn. In planning a research project, identify gaps in knowledge and endeavour to fill those gaps, otherwise the research might not contribute much to the existing body of knowledge. To be meaningful, the investigator must clearly identify the problem statement and the purpose statement.

The methodology includes the design, sample and methods of measurement. The research design is also known as a blueprint that outlines the activities to be undertaken throughout the research process. For instance, in research employing a quantitative approach, the design ensures control over those factors that could interfere with the validity of the findings. Research directed to determining whether one factor causes a specific result tends to occur within a laboratory setting where the environment can be controlled. The sample is the group of subjects selected to participate in the research. Typically, a sample is expected to be representative, that is, to reflect the salient characteristics of the population for which the results may be generalized. Careful attention is directed to identifying the object of interest and how that object will be measured (e.g. items on a survey or observation of actions).

Polit and Hungler (1999) describe ethical considerations that must be addressed when human subjects participate in research activities. They identify three principles (*ibid.*, pp. 134–140):

- **The principle of beneficence** includes freedom from harm and freedom from exploitation.
- **The principle of respect for human dignity** includes the right to self-determinism and the right to full disclosure.
- **The principle of justice** includes the right to fair treatment and the right to privacy, which refers to anonymity and confidentiality.

Anonymity and confidentiality are integral to all research activity:

> *Anonymity occurs when even the researcher cannot link a participant with the information for that person ... [and] a promise of confidentiality to participants is a pledge that any information that the participant provides will not be publicly reported in a manner that identifies the participant or made accessible to parties other than those involved in the research.* (ibid., p. 139)

Research participants also have a right to be fully informed about the purpose of the research, what their involvement entails, the risks and benefits, and the option of voluntarily agreeing to participate or decline participation without any adverse affects on their relationship with the researcher. Responding to a survey is deemed to be consent to participate whereas individuals who participate in an interview sign an informed consent form. University and health-care organizations usually have formal ethics review committees to assess the adherence to ethical principles for any research involving human subjects.

Importantly, each problem may be investigated through a quantitative or qualitative methodology. Quantitative research tends to be concerned with the collection and analysis of objective data in numerical form. Thus, it is possible to collect large volumes of data and seek representative samples for generalizing from the findings. The researcher often collects data through a survey or questionnaire. Conversely, qualitative research is open to collecting and analysing data in many different forms. The qualitative researcher seeks to explore concepts from the perspective of those individuals best informed about the topic. The researcher collects data through face-to-face interviews in a setting natural to the participant, hence this research is considered subjective. The sample size is often small because the researcher seeks to pursue the concept in some 'depth'. Therefore it is critical that the components of the research process are linked through an appropriate philosophical base that underpins the problem, the research design and research methods as well as the interpretation of the research findings.

The final step in conducting research entails knowledge utilization, essentially sharing the findings with others and using the information to inform practice. This task can be achieved by presenting research findings at local, national and international conferences. Furthermore, depending on the research undertaken, researchers often present the findings to the individuals who participated in the research. For instance, when employees participate in various research activities (e.g. surveys or interviews), senior administrators often request feedback on how the organization responded compared to other participants. Occasionally, it is not possible to separate one organization's response from another, but the researcher is willing to share the findings from the research activity. However, the dissemination of research findings is one aspect in achieving the goal of evidence-based health care.

CONDUCTING A SOUND LITERATURE REVIEW

A literature review is a critical step in the research process. Its timing may depend on whether the researcher is conducting a quantitative or qualitative research study. Some qualitative researchers deliberately avoid conducting an in-depth literature search at the start of their research; this is to avoid biasing their thinking on a topic.

Burns and Grove (2001) explain that literature refers to 'all written sources relevant to the topic you have selected' (p. 107) and that this literature may be identified as primary or secondary sources. Primary sources are documents written by the individual or group of individuals who originally identified the idea, conducted the research or developed the theory. Secondary sources are documents that cite the work of other individuals. In secondary sources a writer is often paraphrasing original primary sources, so there is considerable opportunity for misunderstandings. Consequently, primary sources are preferable to secondary sources.

The purpose of a literature review is to identify what is known and not known about a concept or phenomenon (Polit and Hungler, 1999). By noting what information is lacking on a topic, the reviewer establishes a gap that can be filled through research. Furthermore, the reviewer notes what theoretical knowledge exists as well as the support, or lack of support, for the proposed theories. The reviewer also delineates the methods used in conducting research and assesses the findings from each method to determine the strengths and weaknesses of various methods. From the literature review, researchers identify and refine the specific focus of a concept to be pursued and the appropriate methods for adding to the current body of knowledge on a specific topic.

Given the cyclical nature of some topics, it may be necessary to conduct a literature review that covers a long period of time. Focus on obtaining the seminal work – original work on a concept – or landmark studies – key stages in the development of a concept – rather than restricting your review to a period of years (Burns and Grove, 2001). Furthermore, a literature review is deemed *complete* when the reviewer notes that no new references are surfacing; this is often called the saturation point. When writing a literature review for a research proposal, include only relevant references that provide an objective perspective on the topic. Nurses doing research routinely use the following indexes and databases:

- The International Nursing Index
- The Cumulative Index to Nursing and Allied Health Literature (CINAHL)
- A Bibliography of Nursing Literature (Royal College of Nursing)
- The Database of Abstracts of Reviews of Effectiveness (DARE)
- The NHS Economic Evaluation Database
- The Health Technology Assessment Database
- Index Medicus
- Cochrane Library (CD-ROM and online)
- Psychological Abstracts.

Numerous electronic databases are now available, easily accessed by computer all around the world. And it is relatively straightforward to obtain copies of specific articles, because many full-text documents can be downloaded from the internet. The difficult task is to specify the keywords central to your area of interest, remaining open to various synonyms and spellings without being sidetracked down extraneous avenues. Reference management software can help with the literature review; two examples are ProCite and EndNote. It is reasonable and relatively easy to limit your search to a meaningful collection of references. If you are identifying too many references using a Boolean search, you could restrict your search to a specific language and to publications within a specific time frame. The World Wide Web is also a source for relevant articles that provide information about the development of a concept as well as research designs, measurement methods and statistical procedures. There are many search engines that help to locate articles on the web; Google is very widely used.

The Cochrane Collaboration supports the Cochrane Library, a database of research evidence available on CD-ROM or online. The National Health Service Centre for Research Dissemination is based at York University; it conducts systematic reviews of health-related research and disseminates its findings. The Department of Health recognizes the need to assess the quality of new evidence and to provide an audit mechanism. To achieve these goals, it established the National Institute for Clinical Excellence (NICE) in 1999. The goal of NICE is to appraise evidence and health-care technologies and to foster the creation and dissemination of evidence-based guidelines and standards for the delivery of care. Furthermore, the Department of Health created the Commission for Health Improvement (CHI) in 2000 to monitor the implementation of standards and, when necessary, to inspect situations where there is a major system failure. Through these initiatives, the Department of Health demonstrates commitment to supporting future research and development within health services.

SOME IMPORTANT WEBSITES FOR HEALTH-CARE INFORMATION

- Cochrane Library: www.update-software.com/ccweb/cochrane/cdsr.htm
- Cochrane Effective Practice and Organization of Care Group (EPOC): www.epoc.uottawa.ca
- The Department of Health: www.doh.gov.uk
- The National Health Service Centre for Reviews and Dissemination: www.york.ac.uk/inst/crd/welcome.htm
- EndNote: www.endnote.com
- Google: www.google.com
- ProCite: www.procite.com
- Qualitative Methods Network: www.iphrp.salford.ac.uk/cochrane/homepage.htm

SPECIAL ISSUES OF JOURNALS

Journal editors occasionally devote an entire issue to one topic. A recent issue of the *Canadian Journal of Nursing Research* focuses on research into older people. McWilliam, the guest editor, writes, 'A cross-section of national and international work, collectively these papers provide an overview of nursing's multifaceted attention to enhancing the health and life of older people' (McWilliam, 2003, p. 3). Writers contributing to this issue demonstrate the use of qualitative approaches and quantitative analysis strategies as well as a systematic literature review and synthesis. For example, Phinney and Wallhagen (2003) advance evidence-based nursing specific to enhancing the health and life of older people who have type-2 diabetes. In another article, Ward-Griffin *et al.* (2003) discuss relationships between families and nurses specific to residents in a long-term care facility. A final example is the systematic literature review of Peacock and Forbes (2003) looking at interventions for caregivers of persons with dementia; it focuses on the strong studies that could contribute to evidence-based decisions on the well-being of caregivers.

However you carry out your literature search, adopt a diligent and systematic approach to recording your findings. A thorough literature review consumes considerable time and energy as you find, select and document articles of interest. Carefully identify the essential information on key references as it will help you to retrace your steps and engenders an organized approach to the literature. For each reference, note the authors, the publication date and the title of the journal article or the book chapter. For journal articles note the volume number, issue number and page numbers; for books note the names of any editors, the book title, relevant page numbers, the state or country of publication and the name of the publisher. The next step is critical analysis of your selected literature.

Activity

- Select a topic of interest to you. Identify the keywords that you would use to conduct a thorough literature search. Compare your list with a relevant library index. You could ask a librarian to help you.
- Identify a concept of interest for a paper you will write during your course. Develop an outline of this paper and use your outline to obtain primary sources to support its development.
- Write your reference list using an appropriate reference format.

ESSENTIAL ASPECTS OF A CRITICAL APPRAISAL

Critical appraisal requires careful reviewing of information before making a judgement on its value. Burns and Grove (2001) suggest that 'an intellectual critique of research involves a systematic, unbiased, careful examination of all aspects of a study to judge the merits, limitations, meaning, and significance based on previous research experience and knowledge of the topic' (p. 663). When you are reviewing an article to support the conduct of a research study or to implement a change in practice, your goal is to arrive at an objective assessment of that article.

Burns and Grove (2001) give five steps for critiquing quantitative research: comprehension, comparison, analysis, evaluation and conceptual clustering. They explain the complex process of conducting a critique and note that baccalaureate-prepared individuals should be able to achieve the steps of comprehension and comparison. Comprehension is typically the first step in critically appraising an article or report. If you are new to research and critiquing, note the terminology and recognize that many terms have a unique meaning. It is the responsibility of the researcher to ensure that terms with specific meanings are clearly defined in their article.

SQ3R

SQ3R stands for survey, question, read, recall and review. It is often recommended to students as a good way to begin a critical appraisal process. Here are the five aspects in more detail:

- **Survey**: start by scanning or skimming the article to find out what the text has to say that is relevant to your needs.
- **Question**: think of questions you would like the text to answer to meet your specific needs.
- **Read**: read only as much of the text as you need for your questions to be answered
- **Recall**: stop reading for a moment and make notes on the main points you have read, using your own words not the author's words.
- **Review**: leave your notes for a while then come back and check that you still understand them; see whether they answer your original questions.

The purpose of taking notes is to increase your attention while you're reading, not to reproduce large sections of the text. Keep your needs firmly in mind when you're reading; don't be sidetracked by other issues.

Related to SQ3R is the idea of reading the abstract and the conclusion before working through the article from start to finish. This heightens your awareness of the key findings and alerts you to salient points in the article. Look for headings and subheadings and use them as signposts for your reading. For instance, when you see headings such as Background, Theoretical Framework, Methods, Sample, Findings, Discussion, you will appreciate the organization of the information. Furthermore, you will soon become skilled at recognizing when a researcher does not include pertinent information in one of those sections. As you read, you begin the process of critiquing the article. Thus, you ask yourself many questions about the work's clarity and comprehensiveness, the logical development of ideas, and how the pieces of information relate to each other. Publishers often restrict the number of words or pages in the articles they publish, so writers are challenged to explain their research as effectively as possible within these restrictions.

In the comparison step, you relate what the researcher is reporting to the ideal situation. This requires you to have a fairly good grasp of the research process. Consult a textbook that explains the research process and how to critique research articles. Polit and Hungler (1999) and Burns and Grove (2001) provide step-by-step guides on doing a critique. For instance, if you know about ethical requirements when human subjects take part in research, it will prompt you to look for a statement acknowledging the rights of participants and how the researchers accommodated them. Also, you will soon recognize the different sampling procedures for quantitative and qualitative methods and readily identify that the researcher is providing sufficient information in a few words. Many words have unique meanings in a research context and you will learn to use terms correctly.

It takes time and commitment to become skilled at critical appraisal. Your critical-thinking skills are valuable as you raise questions about what you're reading and you wonder about what is and isn't written. As you get better at appraising other people's research articles, you should get better at criticizing your own work. The Critical Appraisal Skills Programme (CASP) has a useful website on critical appraisal skills; you can find it at www.phru.nhs.uk/casp/casp.htm.

Activity

- Define what critical appraisal means to you.
- Identify an area where you could improve your critical appraisal skills. Determine one way in which you could improve that skill.
- Review a chapter in a research text about critiquing a research article. Note the different questions and comments on how to critique a quantitative research report and a qualitative research report.
- Read a research article and identify its strengths and weaknesses.

BASIC STATISTICS REPORTED IN A RESEARCH ARTICLE

To judge the value of a study, you will need to understand statistics. Assess whether or not the data have been interpreted accurately and fairly. The basic principles of statistics are not difficult to understand. Even a novice can be alert to how they may be misused. For instance, using your critical-thinking skills, assess the extent to which the findings appear reasonable. Do the figures in tables match the figures in the accompanying text?

Researchers rarely present fraudulent results. Fraudulent results mean that the statistical analyses and any conclusions based on them are worthless. It is difficult to tell whether results are fabricated, but you may be suspicious if the calculations appear too neat. You may also be curious about data collection procedures and doubt their authenticity. Fortunately, very few researchers exaggerate their findings. It is just as important to understand why something doesn't work as to know that something does work.

Research results may be interpreted in a variety of ways, depending on the reason behind the work. For example, a manager may wish to show where savings in educational costs can be achieved whereas an educator may wish to demonstrate a need for further investment. The two conclusions, based on the same results, may reflect the selective or perhaps biased interpretations of the two individuals, but not false results.

A simple example of biased interpretation can occur in the choice of presenting an average as a mean, median or mode. The mean is obtained by summing all scores and dividing the total by the number of scores. If you have spent £3, £4, £45, £7 and £5 on a set of presents, the total spent is £64 and the mean amount spent per present is £64/5 = £12.80. The mean is the most commonly used average. It can give a misleading impression because it can be distorted by one or two atypical results. Here one of the presents cost £45 and it has distorted the mean. The median is the middle result if you arrange all the scores in numerical order. In this example the median amount spent per present is £5. The median is a useful average in situations where you have one or two extreme results. The mode is the score that occurs most frequently. If someone asked you how long it usually took you to travel to work, you might think like this:

> *If I catch the bus, which I usually do, it takes me half an hour. If I get a lift in, it will take less time. If I miss the bus and have to wait for the next bus, it will take me 50 minutes. But most days I catch the bus, so the best answer is half an hour.*

Half an hour is the mode. It is important to know whether the effect of intervention is caused by chance. Many research studies attempt to show a correlation between different variables, such as a relationship between people's age and their willingness to accept a new therapy. Statistics assist researchers to report that the effect is unlikely to have been caused by chance. Therefore, in reading research reports, you look for evidence that the researcher has subjected the results to a statistical test. Researchers carefully report the statistical analyses they have completed and they generally explain why they chose some statistical tests instead of others.

In some research it is possible to demonstrate that a cause-and-effect relationship has been established. Only true experimental research designs can discover if there is genuinely cause and effect. True experimental research has to meet several criteria: manipulation of the independent variable, also called the treatment or experimental intervention; using a control group; and randomly assigning subjects to the treatment group or the control group. Only when these criteria are met is it possible to demonstrate cause and effect. Read research reports to determine whether researchers inappropriately attribute cause and effect to their findings. For example, based on a survey, a researcher may state that smokers have lower salaries than non-smokers. What does this imply? Does it mean that smokers are less likely to be promoted, that people smoke because they are undervalued at work, or that smoking and lower salaries are both influenced by another factor not mentioned in the survey, a factor such as age or educational qualifications?

You will need an extensive knowledge of statistics if you are diligently going to assess research findings. However, some mistakes in reporting findings are common and easy to detect. Sometimes researchers attempt to demonstrate results when their figures have no numerical meaning. There are different kinds of scale and each has its correct usage. For instance, if a researcher has placed the weights of infants in rank order from the lightest to the heaviest, they are using an ordinal scale in units of weight, such as kilograms or pounds and ounces.

Box 5.1

Key concepts in research

- **Basic research**: concerned with generating new knowledge, learning, and finding truth.
- **Concept**: a mental image or generalization of an object, property or event that is derived from individual perceptual experience. Concepts can be concrete (specific to time or place) or abstract (independent of time and place). Concepts are the building blocks of theory.
- **Cross-sectional study**: a study that examines groups of subjects in various stages of development at one point in time with the intention of inferring trends.
- **Data**: pieces of information or facts that are collected in a research study. The word 'data' is plural whereas the word 'datum' is singular.
- **Epistemology**: theory of knowledge.
- **Hypothesis**: a formal statement of the expected relationship between two or more variables in a specific population.
- **Knowledge**: an awareness or perception of reality acquired through learning or investigation.
- **Laboratory study**: the study of subjects in a special environment that has been created by the researchers.
- **Limitations**: theoretical or methodological shortcomings that may limit the generalizability of the research findings.
- **Qualitative study**: a systematic, interactive, subjective approach to research that is concerned with in-depth descriptions of people or events. Data are collected through such methods as unstructured interviews and participant observation. Qualitative research endeavours to give meaning to the phenomena under study.
- **Quantitative research**: a formal, objective, systematic process that is concerned with numbers and other data that can be converted into numbers. This approach intends to describe relationships and, specifically, to test cause-and-effect relationships among variables.
- **Sample**: a subset of the population that is chosen to represent the population and used to make generalizations about the population under study.
- **Science**: the systematic and objective study of phenomena, based traditionally on observation, experiment and measurement. Science also refers to a body of knowledge that includes research findings, tested theories, scientific principles and laws for a discipline.
- **Survey**: a type of non-experimental research that focuses on obtaining information about the status quo of some situation.

Data are often collected through questionnaires or personal interviews; surveys have the advantage of obtaining information from a large sample of respondents.

- **Target population**: the group of people or objects to which the researcher wishes to generalize the findings of a study.
- **Theory**: an integrated set of defined concepts, definitions and propositions about phenomena. The purpose of theories is to describe, explain, predict and/or control the phenomenon of interest.

Activity

- Select a research report from the literature. Identify any words that you do not understand. Identify any key words used in the article that the authors did not define.
- Using any nursing research text, define the terms 'conceptual' and 'operational definitions' for key ideas used in your paper.
- Look at the key concepts in this chapter and select three that you do not understand. Using nursing research texts, read about these three words to elucidate their meanings in a research context.

SUMMARY

To summarize, the E-BP movement is moving forward at a rapid pace. The medical and nursing professions are at the forefront in seeking evidence to support their practice. Debates in the literature about what constitutes evidence are essential to ensure there is a common understanding of E-BP, its related concepts and eventually practice guidelines. With its goal of providing the best possible health care for all individuals, many people hope this movement will continue. Research is a systematic and rigorous activity. This chapter emphasized the importance of a thorough literature review; you will be expected to do this when you write a paper. Moreover, before writing your paper, you will use your skills of critical analysis to review the literature you have selected. It takes time and commitment to develop these skills.

Key points ▶

1 The E-BP movement is moving forward and challenging all disciplines to remain current and effective in delivering care to the public.
2 Research is a systematic, rigorous process of inquiry to explore specific concepts or phenomena for validating or refining current knowledge or for creating new knowledge on those concepts or phenomena.
3 The terms used to explain research tend to have unique meanings; readers should make sure they understand these unique meanings.

4   E-BP refers to practice founded on sound research findings.
5   A well-conducted literature review should uncover relevant articles as a starting point for new research. It requires patience, organization, energy and attention to detail.
6   Computers have made it easier to do literature searches.
7   Technology increases the chances of obtaining information in a timely fashion. Government documents are readily available on the web.
8   Critical appraisal skills are essential for selecting and using literature appropriately.

REFERENCES

Angel, B. F., Duffey, M. and Belyea, M. (2000) An evidence-based project for evaluating strategies to improve knowledge acquisition and critical-thinking performance in nursing students. *Journal of Nursing Education*, **39**(5), 219–229.

Briggs, A. (1972) *Report of the Committee on Nursing*. HMSO, London.

Burns, N. and Grove, S. K. (2001) *The Practice of Nursing Research: Conduct, Critique, and Utilization*, 4th edn. W. B. Saunders, London.

Caramanica, L., Maljanian, R., McDonald, D., Kelly-Taylor, S., MacRae, J. B. and Beland, D. K. (2002) Evidence-based nursing practice, Part 1: A hospital and university collaborative. *Journal of Nursing Administration*, **32**(1), 27–30.

Cochrane, A. L. (1972) *Effectiveness and Efficiency: Random Reflections on Health Services*. Nuffield Provincial Hospitals Trust, London.

Cooper, H., Carlisle, C., Gibbs, T. and Watkins, C. (2001) Developing an evidence base for interdisciplinary learning: a systematic review. *Journal of Advanced Nursing*, **35**(2), 228–237.

Davies, D. (2003) Towards a learning society. In: *Theory and Practice of Nursing: An Integrated Approach to Caring Practice*, 2nd edn (ed. Basford, L. and Slevin, O.). Nelson Thornes, Cheltenham, Glos., pp. 120–138.

DiCenso, A. and Cullum, N. (1998) Implementing evidence-based nursing: some misconceptions. *Evidence-Based Nursing*, **1**(2), 38–40.

Estabrooks, C. A. (1998) Will evidence-based nursing practice make practice perfect? *Canadian Journal of Nursing Research*, **30**(1), 15–36.

French, P. (2002) What is the evidence on evidence-based nursing? An epistemological concern. *Journal of Advanced Nursing*, **37**(3), 250–257.

Freshwater, D. (2003) Clinical supervision and leadership. In: *Theory and Practice of Nursing: An Integrated Approach to Caring Practice*, 2nd edn (ed. Basford, L. and Slevin, O.). Nelson Thornes, Cheltenham, Glos., pp. 112–119.

Hunt, J. (2001) Research into practice: the foundation for evidence-based care. *Cancer Nursing*, **24**(2), 78–87.

Jennings, B. M. and Loan, L. A. (2001) Misconceptions among nurses about evidence-based practice. *Journal of Nursing Scholarship*, **33**(2), 121–127.

Kitson, A. (2002) Recognizing relationships: reflections on evidence-based practice. *Nursing Inquiry*, **9**(3), 179–186.

Kitson, A., Harvey, G. and McCormack, B. (1998) Enabling the implementation of evidence-based practice: a conceptual framework. *Quality of Health Care*, 7, 149–158.

Maljanian, R., Caramanica, L., Kelly-Taylor, S., MacRae, J. B. and Beland, D. K. (2002) Evidence-based nursing practice, Part 2: Building skills through research roundtables. *Journal of Nursing Administration*, **32**(2), 85–90.

McCormack, B., Kitson, A., Harvey, G., Rycroft-Malone, J., Titchen, A. and Seers, K. (2002) Getting evidence into practice: the meaning of 'context'. *Journal of Advanced Nursing*, **38**(1), 94–104.

McWilliam, C. (2003) Advancing the contributions of gerontological nursing research. *Canadian Journal of Nursing Research*, **35**(4), 3–5.

Mulhall, A. (1998) Nursing, research, and the evidence. *Evidence-Based Nursing*, **1**, 4–6.

Peacock, S. C. and Forbes, D. A. (2003) Interventions for caregivers of persons with dementia: a systematic review. *Canadian Journal of Nursing Research*, **35**(4), 88–107.

Pearson, A. (2003) Clinical effectiveness: an evidence base for practice. In: *Theory and Practice of Nursing: An Integrated Approach to Caring Practice*, 2nd edn (ed. Basford, L. and Slevin, O.). Nelson Thornes, Cheltenham, Glos., pp. 320–327.

Phinney, A. and Wallhagen, M. (2003) Recognizing and understanding the symptoms of type 2 diabetes. *Canadian Journal of Nursing Research*, **35**(4), 108–124.

Polit, D. F. and Hungler, B. P. (1999) *Nursing Research Principles and Methods*, 6th edn. Lippincott, Philadelphia.

Qualitative Methods Network (1999) Report on Rome Workshop, November 1999. Available from www.iphrp.salford.ac.uk/cochrane/stpress.htm.

Retsas, A. (2000) Barriers to using research evidence in nursing practice. *Journal of Advanced Nursing*, **31**(3), 599–606.

Sackett, D. L., Rosenberg, W. M. C., Gray, M. J. A. and Haynes, R. B. (1996) Evidence-based medicine: what it is and what it isn't. *British Medical Journal*, **312**, 71–72.

Senge, P. M. (1990) *The Fifth Discipline: The Art and Practice of the Learning Organization*. Doubleday Currency, New York.

Senge, P. M. (1996) Leading learning organizations: the bold, the powerful, and the invisible. In: *The Leader of the Future: New Visions, Strategies, and Practices for the Next Era* (ed. Hesslebein, F., Goldsmith, M. and Beckhard R.). Jossey-Bass, San Francisco, pp. 41–57.

Stone, P. A., Curran, C. R. and Bakken, S. (2002) Economic evidence for evidence-based practice. *Journal of Nursing Scholarship*, **34**(3), 277–282.

Ward-Griffin, C., Bol, N., Hay, K. and Dashnay, I. (2003) Relationships between families and registered nurses in long-term care facilities: a critical analysis. *Canadian Journal of Nursing Research*, **35**(4), 150–174.

FURTHER READING

Davies, P. (1999) What is evidence-based education? *British Journal of Educational Studies*, **47**(2), 108–121.

Flemming, K. (1998) Asking answerable questions. *Evidence-Based Nursing*, **1**(2), 36–37.

Forbes, D. and Clark, K. (2003). The Cochrane Library can answer your nursing care effectiveness questions. *Canadian Journal of Nursing*, **35**(3), 18–25.

French, P. (1999) The development of evidence-based nursing. *Journal of Advanced Nursing*, **29**(1), 72–78.

Harvey, G., Loftus-Hills, A., Rycroft-Malone, J., Titchen, A., Kitson, A., McCormack, B. and Seers, K. (2002) Getting evidence into practice: the role and function of facilitation. *Journal of Advanced Nursing*, **37**(6), 577–588.

Ingersoll, G. L. (2000). Evidence-based nursing: what it is and what it isn't. *Nursing Outlook*, **48**(4), 151–152.

Website

EBN Online: http://ebn.bmjjournals.com

COMMUNICATING EFFECTIVELY WITH OLDER PEOPLE

6

Leslie Vaala

OBJECTIVES

- Define communication in the context of health care.
- Discuss the need for effective communication when caring for older people.
- Discuss the use of technology for communicating more effectively.
- Describe the importance of communicating within and between professional groups to enable more effective care.
- Discuss the need to keep and maintain patient and client records.

INTRODUCTION

Communication is essential to all aspects of care, including organization and therapeutics. Most failures of care delivery are attributed to a lack of effective communication. Effective communication is vital to high-quality health care and is a core skill for all health-care professionals. Most people interact through forms of communication on an everyday basis, but in a health-care setting the emphasis is significantly different in that it embraces a range of skills, knowledge and professional frameworks. Although the knowledge and skill base are generic, they need to be extended and applied to the specific needs of older people, particularly when they have physical, mental or social limitations.

Activity

Before starting your reading, orient yourself with Mary's experience. Reflect in your learning journal some of the issues that relate to poor and improper communication within Mary's case. When you have completed this chapter, you can then go back to these journal entries and do a self-assessment exercise on your previous awareness and knowledge of communication when caring for older people.

EXPLAINING COMMUNICATION

The term 'communication' covers just about any interaction with another individual. It includes the sharing of information, ideas and feelings between people. A complex phenomenon, it is often broken down into component parts to make it easier to understand.

The communication chain

Communication is a two-way process. When you communicate, you perceive the other person's responses and react with your own thoughts and feelings. Your behaviour is generated by your internal responses to what you see and hear. It is only by paying attention to the other person that you have any idea about what to say or do next. In one-to-one communication, your partner is also responding to your behaviour in the same way.

People who interact effectively with other people are said to have good communication skills. The keys to successful communication are being aware of how you're communicating, possessing a range of skills, and building up your experience and confidence. To ensure your communication is effective, you need to recognize the different forms of communication and use them appropriately. Communication is more than the words we say. It is thought that over 55% of the impact of any communication is determined by body language. These two types of communication, words and body language, are often known as verbal communication and non-verbal communication. Here are the five forms of communication:

- **language**: words that are spoken or written (e.g. English, Somali, Urdu) or signed (e.g. British Sign Language).
- **speech**: sounds that make up the words.
- **sensory contact**: any communication through the senses (seeing, hearing, smelling, touching).
- **body language**: gestures, facial expressions, postures and physical distance from other people.
- **activities**: interaction based on sharing activities such as arts and crafts, sport, music and drama.

Language and active listening

Health-care professionals need good language skills in speech and comprehension. They need language and listening skills for communicating effectively in many different ways: talking one-to-one with a patient, a colleague or on the telephone; talking to a group; or participating in group discussions. As well as spoken language, the use of written language is a vital part of effective communication. Legible, comprehensive, easily understood written records require effective communication skills.

Professionals need to be 'active listeners' to hear and understand what patients and colleagues are telling them. An active listener

- gives full attention to the speaker;
- makes appropriate eye contact with the speaker, not staring too hard but with 'soft eyes';
- lets the other person speak without interrupting;
- hears the words the speaker says;
- responds to the non-verbal messages conveyed by body language;

- concentrates on understanding the messages;
- encourages the speaker to continue, by nodding and giving encouraging words and signs at appropriate places;
- responds in an appropriate way.

An active listener is genuinely interested in hearing what someone has to say. A health-care professional who listens actively will be able to interpret the patient's meaning and translate it into something that will improve the care of that patient. Health-care professionals need to have highly developed active listening skills. However, this type of listening can be a challenge because it requires concentration. We cannot actively listen to everyone all the time, but there are times when we need to ensure that we listen carefully to what patients tell us, and interpret what they are expressing correctly by seeing things from their perspective, not our own.

What stops you listening to older patients? Do you have active listening skills? If not, bear in mind that failure to listen actively is a communication barrier. You may not be able to break the communication barrier single-handedly, even if you are good at active listening, but there are three ways you can help:

- **relaxing**: if you are tense, your patient will sense this tension and it will be more difficult for both of you to communicate effectively.
- **making and taking time**: making time now may save time in the long run, even if heavy workloads tempt you to do otherwise.
- **feeling confident**: know that you can communicate effectively with the patient in some way.

Turn-taking skills

Taking turns is an important skill in conversation. It is an unspoken rule that we have come to expect. An important aspect of conversation is feedback from the listener to the speaker and the continuation of this communication loop. If turn-taking is not properly observed, people may be talked at or not responded to. This may make them feel uneasy. Aim to develop turn-taking skills yourself and in your patients. Turn-taking encourages feedback, and feedback is essential to effective communication.

The singer and the song

Feelings and emotions are conveyed by words and how we say them:

- tone of voice, e.g. harsh, bright, flat
- pitch, e.g. high or low
- volume
- speed
- emphasis on particular words
- pauses
- gestures
- facial expression

- intonation, i.e. the melody and rhythm of speech
- other body language such as eye contact, body position, physical movement or lack of it.

Just as health-care professionals should be looking for signs that show how a patient is feeling, so patients are also able to interpret the health-care professional's thoughts and emotions.

Many of us speak slowly to older people, believing it will help them to hear and understand more clearly. In one study of a group of people aged between 65 and 88, researchers found that when speech rates were slowed to 60% of normal rate, sentence comprehension increased significantly (Schmitt and McCroskey, 1981). However, understanding also increased significantly when speech rates were speeded up to 140% of normal speed. The researchers speculated that the speeded-up voice was novel enough to increase older listeners' attention to the experimental task, thereby resulting in higher comprehension scores. But whatever the speed, the clarity of the spoken word is the important factor in facilitating understanding.

Speech

The sounds of our words are produced by finely coordinated movements of the jaw, tongue, soft palate, larynx and breath.

Sensory and non-verbal communication (body language)

Sensory communication is communication involving the senses of hearing, sight, touch and smell. Illness and ageing often affect older people's sensory input. If you would like to know more about this topic, you could read *Nursing in Nursing Homes* (Nazarko, 1995). There is also information about hearing and visual impairment later in this chapter. People communicate through touch and presence (i.e. how close they stand to each other). Some older people who are frail and vulnerable welcome the comfort of an arm around the shoulder or a squeeze of the hand. However, for others, physical closeness, although meant to offer reassurance and support, may seem intrusive and patronizing. How do you know your patients' preferences about physical closeness?

We need to be sensitive to people's feelings. In addition, we have to be careful that physical contact is not misinterpreted, particularly when we are alone with patients. On occasions when physical contact is necessary, the patient should be given an explanation of what is being done and treated gently and respectfully; examples of this are during an examination, washing, dressing or giving treatment. You might find it helpful to read *Practitioner–Client Relationships and the Prevention of Abuse* (UKCC, 1999). Remember that different cultures have different conventions about body space, touch and proximity.

The way people position and move their bodies when interacting with others gives clear signals about how they are feeling, even if they are not aware of it. Here are some examples of body language:

- gestures
- facial expressions
- posture
- body positions.

Gestures include shrugging, waving, nodding, shaking the head and giving a thumbs-up sign. When you choose a posture, aim to position yourself face-to-face and on the same level as your patient, especially if the person is hard of hearing or language-impaired.

When people are comfortable with each other and communicating well, they often unconsciously copy each other's body language. This behaviour is called mirroring, which helps to create a rapport. Mirroring a patient's body language may improve communication. However, beware of mimicking the patient. Nobody likes to feel they are being ridiculed.

Facial expressions

Six core facial expressions exist in most cultures. They correspond to the emotions of happiness, surprise, fear, sadness, anger, and disgust or contempt. You can probably instantly picture each of these expressions in your mind's eye, but they can be deceptive or harder to recognize when people are feeling frail and vulnerable. This is revealed in the following statement in a formal complaint by a patient's relative: 'I thought, I'm not going to let her see what I'm feeling. I didn't like her at all, so I just smiled at her, but inside I was very angry'.

Effective interaction

Using body language effectively can greatly enhance communication with patients, particularly if they have difficulties with verbal communication. Be aware of your body language in your interactions with older people. Greet them with a smile, making appropriate eye contact and welcoming gestures. Once the conversation is under way, demonstrate that you are actively listening:

- Show interest through eye contact.
- Show recognition and friendliness in your facial expressions.
- Show closeness through your body position in relation to the other person's.
- Show empathy by naturally mirroring the other person's gestures and body position.
- Show openness by leaning forward slightly, with your arms and legs unfolded.
- Show calmness through relaxed muscles and posture.

Figure 6.1 shows a health-care professional communicating with an older person using touch and eye contact.

Interacting effectively is often not that simple. When you are busy and interacting with the same people continually, it is easy to lapse and be tempted to take short cuts. Although a friendly demeanour, warmth

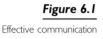

Figure 6.1

Effective communication

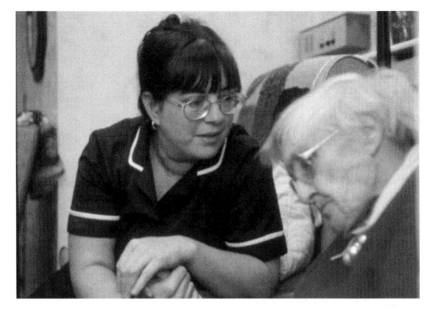

and a degree of personal contact can be helpful in establishing and maintaining effective communication, sometimes these actions are not enough:

> *Joyce, a care worker with many years of experience, comes into the room. She approaches Elsie from behind her chair, touches her on the arm and says cheerfully: 'Time for lunch now, Elsie. It's roast chicken, one of your favourites. I hope there'll be enough to go round. Are you ready to go? We don't want it to get cold.' Elsie looks a little startled and says: 'I am not feeling cold, thank you.' (Adapted from Knocker, 1998)*

Elsie has dementia, but the difficulties she had coping with Joyce's greeting are also likely to be encountered by other older people. You may have noted the following points:

- Joyce gives Elsie no warning of her approach and makes physical contact before checking, through eye contact and speech, that Elsie is aware of her presence. For a person with dementia, the initial approach is particularly important, as it can take time to engage or connect. Here Elsie only really tunes in to Joyce's last few words. If the person with dementia is not ready to hear what you are saying, you are likely to confuse them and communication is hindered. If Elsie had impaired hearing or even if she could hear perfectly but had just woken up, she could be similarly not ready to hear and be confused. Understanding may also be hampered in either case if there is too much background noise, such as from the television or other people talking.
- Joyce may be speaking too rapidly and trying to say too many things at once, all too common when in a rush or feeling stressed. Shorter

sentences are better, with a maximum length of seven words. If seven words are too many, try five. Use simple words. Check that the patient has tuned in to each statement before moving on to the next one; this is particularly important if the patient has dementia.

- Getting the body language right is also vital. Communication is more effective if you are at the same level as the person you are talking to. Standing above the person may make them feel intimidated. Make eye contact. Use your eyes to establish trust and communicate warmth.
- Using your hands to make a connection with someone can be a powerful tool, provided you both feel comfortable with the familiarity of touch.

Activity

Go back to Mary's experience and consider how it could have been made better through the use of effective communication skills, if the health care practitioner had communicated with Mary and family or indeed if they had communicated with each other.

Hobbies and activities

Taking part in hobbies or activities often helps people to interact and communicate with each other in a natural, relaxed context. Activities such as art and craft, dance, drama, exercise and music can all provide an opportunity to establish better relationships and understanding through shared experience, thereby increasing the likelihood of meaningful communication. This sort of contact is sometimes called engagement.

Activity

- Having identified the various communication skills, reflect in your learning diary on a clinical situation that could have been made more effective if you or others had been more competent and/or knowledgeable in applying communication skills with older people.
- In the library or on the internet, seek evidence of effective communication skills being used in clinical practice.
- Seek information on service failure in older care settings where the quality of care has been seriously impaired by ineffective communication.

THE NEED TO COMMUNICATE EFFECTIVELY WITH OLDER PEOPLE

Effective communication is an essential part of providing a high standard of care. When good communication is missing, health-care and social services professionals can misunderstand or be ignorant of patients' and carers' needs and expectations; furthermore, patients may not understand their rights and the choices available to them. Along with speech, body language conveys our mood and feelings to other people, but we may be unaware of our body language when interacting with patients. The result can be a mixed message or a misunderstood message. If this misunderstanding causes communication to break down, patients may not receive the treatment or support they need. They may even be put at risk. The health and care sectors are not unique in needing effective communication to provide a good service and minimize inconvenience or distress. How many times have you been delayed on a train, in a plane or in a shopping queue and said to yourself, 'Just what is going on? It wouldn't be so bad if only they'd tell us what's happening!'

Activity

- You can probably think of many occasions when lack of communication has caused you to feel angry or worried. You may even recall times when you failed to communicate effectively with someone and caused them concern. Record these events in your learning diary and critically reflect on them.

When people are vulnerable through illness, through disability or when coping with bereavement, the effects of poor communication can result in more than minor irritation. End-of-life care has a legacy of failing patients and their relatives or friends through ineffective communication that has resulted in patients dying an undignified, humiliating and painful death. Sometimes this is due to the health professionals' own inadequacy in communicating with the dying, so much so that they often use avoidance or communication barrier techniques. When these characteristics are commonly used in clinical practice, this can be detrimental to the health professionals' own health and well-being.

Health-care professionals can become enormously important to someone going into hospital. They are involved in the person's intimate physical and emotional circumstances, and are often their primary source of information, communication and support. Every year the Health Commission publishes a report on formal complaints made about the NHS. Complaints made against NHS staff are mainly to do with communication: the way information is given, staff attitudes, advocacy, guidance and support. The information patients receive about their condition can vary considerably. A survey of discharged patients aged over 65 was conducted in 1997 to investigate their views about the information they received relating to their condition and treatment while in hospital (Smith *et al.*, 1997). Some patients felt they had been kept fully informed and up to date on what was happening to them. They appreciated being told about their prognosis, viewing X-rays and being given literature. Being underinformed caused problems and distress: 'It was like a closed shop and you were left groping around in the dark'. Patients were also unhappy when staff failed to use appropriate language, speaking in terms that went over their heads: 'I was told things I couldn't understand. They told me I'd had a Thompson's. But what's that?' Professionals can also cause patients unnecessary anxiety or even frighten them: 'When I asked my doctor about glaucoma, she said, "You don't want to know about that. It's a nasty disease".'

The survey also showed that the attitudes of the staff could affect patients' views. Some patients felt that the staff had been approachable and allowed them to ask questions; others felt intimidated and undervalued by staff: 'Staff act as though you shouldn't be asking'. A number of patients pointed out their need for reassurance and support: 'You need someone to talk to you to explain what is happening and the feelings you have'.

Activity

Consult your hospital or primary care trust's complaints record. Identify the reasons for complaints with older people. Make a graph indicating these reasons and ascertain whether ineffective communication is part of the complaint.

The way information is given can empower patients to make choices about the care they receive. Health Advisory Service 2000 carried out an independent inquiry into the care of older people on acute wards in general hospitals (Health Advisory Service 2000, 1998). Here are two of its recommendations:

- Older people and their families must be more involved with their care at every stage and in relation to every decision made about their care.
- Patients, their relatives and staff must all take responsibility for assertively challenging negative views about old age and the propensity for ill health, particularly the belief that prospects for recovery are gloomy.

In an executive summary, the same report acknowledges the impact of pressure on staff:

> *Patients, relatives and staff all agree that staff are under considerable pressure from heavy workloads, which directly impact upon the quality of care delivered. Many relatives are dissatisfied with the adequacy of communication from ward teams. Staff are aware of this and feel frustrated that pressures on them may leave insufficient time for communication with patients and their relatives.*

Emotional effects of communication difficulties

People with problems communicating often experience emotional distress caused by loneliness; negative self-image; lack of self-esteem; clinical depression; stress leading to strong emotional reactions such as anger, frustration and anxiety; and boredom. Even day-to-day communication failures can be upsetting. You may have had the experience of feeling that your general practitioner (GP) is not paying attention to you during a surgery visit. When you leave the surgery, you may well feel worse than before you arrived. When your GP listens, you usually feel better. Whether mild or severe, communication problems can result in the individual feeling, and perhaps being, socially excluded to varying degrees. Furthermore, communication problems can cause difficulties with personal relationships, negative reactions from other people, loss of employment opportunities, financial hardship, reduced leisure activities and increased dependency. All of these situations can negatively affect an individual's emotional and psychological well-being.

Incomplete communication prompts making assumptions

Assumptions are based on incomplete or inaccurate communication. We are making an assumption by using the terms 'older person' or 'older patient' as labels in a health-care context. The number of people in the UK older than 65 years is growing, and health and care organizations are beginning to develop ways of managing the increasing demand for services for older people. However, organizations should also be capable of responding flexibly to accommodate people's needs as individuals. We need to be responsive to the enormous variation in the health and fitness of older people. A 75-year-old could be seen as someone who places an inordinate burden on health services, although many people aged 75 are fit and enjoy vigorous sports and leisure activities. Younger people can sometimes forget this. An institutional culture also encourages this attitude.

We all make assumptions based on our knowledge, our previous experiences, other people's opinions and our personal prejudices. Because assumptions are often untested, they can lead to stereotyping and inhibit communication. The following extract illustrates how patients and professionals generally have different assumptions about recovery after a stroke:

> *Studies report differences in patients' and professionals' views of what constitutes recovery. Patients have definite goals and measure recovery in terms of a resumption of previously valued activities. Professionals, on the other hand, view recovery as the return of any discrete movement. Patients accept that they may not regain their pre-stroke functional ability, but won't accept the assessment of the professional, i.e. their prediction of eventual recovery is lower than the patient's own expectations. (Kelson and Ford, 1998)*

These authors report that some professionals had low expectations for patients' recovery after stroke and 'at their most extreme, both patients and carers reported health professionals who painted a very bleak, yet in hindsight, unfounded, outlook on recovery'.

Assumptions about a patient's expected recovery often affect the treatment patients receive from their therapists. For example, many therapists working with aphasic patients have been more pessimistic than either the patient or the patient's spouse, who were equally optimistic. Low expectations can negatively influence the therapeutic relationship and should be overcome in favour of positive assumptions about recovery as far as possible (Gravell, 1988). Professionals often unintentionally cause confusion in older patients and relatives by telling them that they will or will not 'get better'. For example, a professional may tell patients that they will not 'get better' after a stroke. The phrase 'get better' is ambiguous. It can either mean 'make a full recovery' or 'improve from where you are now'.

Even highly professional people with considerable experience sometimes make erroneous assumptions about their patients' attitudes, knowledge and understanding. The following example illustrates the need for effective communication. Many of us judge other people's cognitive abilities by the way they speak or write, or by their voice or body language. But difficulty with expression does not necessarily indicate difficulty with comprehension; difficulty with expression may result from many causes: disease, stroke, invasive operations, and so on. Jean-Dominique Bauby suffered a massive stroke and slipped into a coma from which he emerged paralysed, speechless and able to move only his left eyelid. He recounted his experience in a book, which he dictated by blinking to indicate each letter as the alphabet was repeatedly read to him. Bauby (1997) describes his life as someone with locked-in syndrome:

> We began to discuss locked-in syndrome. Since most victims are abandoned to a vegetable existence, the evolution of the disease is not well understood. All that is known is that if the nervous system makes up its mind to start working again, it does so at the speed of a hair growing from the base of the brain. So it is likely that several years will go by before I can expect to wiggle my toes. In fact it is in my respiratory passages that I can hope for improvement. In the long term, I can hope to eat more normally: that is, without the help of a gastric tube. Eventually perhaps, I could breathe naturally, without a respirator, and muster enough breath to make my vocal cords vibrate.

Active listening

Communicating effectively with older people not only means providing them with useful information, but also hearing what they are saying. Since the ageing process often results in a loss of communication abilities, care staff need to acquire appropriate listening skills. These

Figure 6.2

Active listening

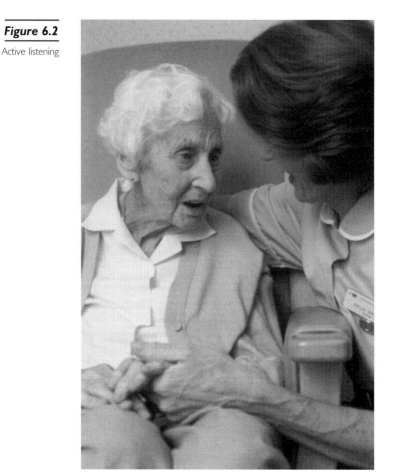

skills are called active listening. Figure 6.2 shows a professional engaging in active listening. Here is another perspective, by Rudyard Kipling:

I keep six honest serving men
(They taught me all I know)
Their names are what and why and when
And how and where and who.

Why do we need to make time to listen?

Covey (1995) suggests that we should 'seek first to understand, then to be understood'. This statement implies the significance of listening to others. Active listening is more than ordinary conversational listening. It is active in the sense that you are devoting your time, full attention and effort to finding out what the other person is saying; you are not just hearing the words, but encountering meaning and feelings. In so many everyday conversations, people don't listen to each other; they wait for their own opportunity to speak, so they can 'exercise their own egos, focusing on themselves and their own thoughts while listening with only half an ear to what the other person is saying, supposedly to them' (Nelson-Jones, 1992).

Effective listening

Features of good listeners
- being non-judgemental
- being accepting
- facing the speaker squarely and having good eye contact
- not interrupting
- allowing silences
- giving time to the speaker
- preventing interruptions
- using body language to reinforce the feeling of encouragement and full attention
- recognizing your own limitations and referring the speaker to other sources of help where appropriate
- smiling warmly when appropriate.

Ellen Newton
Here is an extract from Ellen Newton's diary, *This Bed My Centre*, about her experience in a nursing home:

> *You miss the more intimate things. Someone at hand to laugh at the right moment. Someone to agree or disagree with you. And someone to linger with you over those thousands of uninteresting, so-like-each-other meals. If you are a woman you may long for an intelligent man to talk to, even for a few minutes, to give you a different point of view. These days, your busy GP hasn't five minutes to spare, even to talk about relevant things. Whatever he thinks, he confides to the sister who is with him as he walks out of your room. (Newton, 1980)*

Activity

Reflect on your own style of listening. Are you an active listener? Do you really hear what people say or do you make early judgements? Quietly observe others and assess the level of their listening skills.

What is effective communication with older people?

Effective communication is just as important to individuals with full communication abilities as it is to individuals with speech, language, writing, hearing or other difficulties. For older people generally, effective communication may serve a therapeutic role: it gives them knowledge about their condition, their environment, what other people expect from them, and a sense of influence, usefulness and belonging. It may also allow them to extend themselves beyond their immediate environment and to be better informed about what is happening in the world outside. There are many sources of information for people with communication difficulties and their carers; here are some examples:

- specialist associations such as the Stroke Association (many have websites)
- support groups
- articles, magazines and journals
- voluntary organizations.

Activity

In your library or on the internet, find information about what is currently deemed effective communication with older people.

The right environment

Research in nursing and residential care homes and other institutions has shown the importance of environment in generating and maintaining good communication among staff and between staff and patients (Lubinski *et al.*, 1985). The restrictions imposed by institutional living, lack of privacy in communal spaces and within one's own room, and the negative connotations of being institutionalized can all inhibit communication. An environment that facilitates effective communication has the following characteristics:

- It encourages interchange.
- It values communication.
- It socially reinforces communication.

Research has also identified symptoms of communication-impaired environments:

- There are few opportunities for successful, meaningful communication.
- Individuals are not valued as communication partners.
- Communication is perceived as worthless or useless.
- Rules govern where and when communication takes place, the type of communication and with whom it occurs.
- There is little variety in communication partners.
- There are few or no opportunities to communicate with people outside the setting.
- There are few places for private conversations.
- Staff do not value or reinforce communication among older patients.
- Patients avoid approaches to other patients.
- There are physical problems with the setting, such as shared rooms or noisy communal areas.
- There is obtrusive noise from television, radio and traffic.

To achieve effective communication, you need to be aware that both patient factors and health-care professional factors influence communication with older people. Patient factors include anxiety, sensory deprivation and cautiousness.

Anxiety

Many older people regularly function at a fairly high level of anxiety. For example, the increased stress of a new or unfamiliar situation may lead to intense arousal, impairing the older person's ability to communicate effectively.

Sensory deprivation

A widespread problem for older people is some form of hearing loss. Men are more affected than women and an estimated 30% of older people are impaired by hearing loss. This loss is potentially the most difficult sensory loss for older people and for people of any age. About 80% of older people function with fair to adequate vision.

Cautiousness

Older people tend to make few errors of fact but may regularly fail to provide a complete picture when communicating. For example, when taking a history, the health-care professional must be aware that older people may omit important aspects of their illnesses. Remember that older people might take longer to respond to inquires when being interviewed for information.

When conversing with older people or collecting information from them, health-care professionals will note their tendency to dwell on particular themes. Older people may spend much time complaining of ailments or recounting detailed histories of bodily functions. At a time when friends and loved ones have died and sensory input is decreased, in many ways it is their own body that keeps them company.

Older people may spend considerable time discussing the many losses experienced in later life, such as the loss of friends and loved ones, loss of activities and even loss of self-esteem. Furthermore, many older people agonize over the loss of physical and mental functions, including physical strength, bowel and bladder control, motor functions and especially the ability to regulate their thoughts and emotions. They may express this loss of thinking and emotional regulation as a fear of 'going crazy'. Finally, although older people tend not to be obsessed with approaching death, it is nevertheless a frequent topic of conversation and there are fears of being alone at the end of life.

Two factors that frequently affect health-care professionals' communication with older people are attitudes towards older people and inadequate understanding of ageing.

Attitudes towards older people

It is not unusual to find fears of ageing and death among the younger and middle-aged members of our modern youth-oriented society. Every health-care professional has to acknowledge these fears and personal feelings in order to establish effective communication with the older person.

Understanding of ageing

Each health-care professional must also attempt to separate myths from reality about ageing. Labelling and stereotyping of older people can be a significant communications barrier. For example, images that older people are senile, mentally ill or hypochondriac impede effective communication. Health-care professionals recognize that understanding ageing comes through developing empathy, which is more easily acquired by experience than from textbooks.

TECHNIQUES FOR EFFECTIVE COMMUNICATION WITH OLDER PEOPLE

There are several techniques that can be learned and practised for developing effective communication with older people. These skills begin with an attitude of respect towards older people and focus on verbal and non-verbal messages.

Demonstrate a respectful approach

Most of us need privacy. Sometimes we just need time on our own, away from other people, to think and take stock. At other times we want to do things without fear of anyone coming in or interrupting us. People have the right to privacy whether they are in short- or long-term care. Acknowledging a person's right to privacy is also respectful. Good communication is essential to maintaining appropriate privacy; conversely, poor or inappropriate communication can destroy privacy in terms of

- being on your own;
- not being seen;
- not being overheard.

Here are the opinions of three professionals:

> *I feel that respecting residents' privacy is essential to preserving their sense of self and dignity. In some homes staff talk to residents about really personal details, and there's lots of other people around. You really shouldn't do that. I don't think that many care and support staff in homes get enough education and support in dealing with older people. (Care worker)*
>
> *Some nurses just strip off beds, leaving patients exposed, quite oblivious to their need for privacy. It's not dignified. And they don't talk to them properly. I know some elderly patients can be difficult. Some are very resistant to receiving treatment. I think in nursing you have to get across to patients that what you are doing for them is the right thing. They need to have it explained. (Hospital nurse)*

> *I have very mixed feelings about the general trend to call residents by their first names. It may give out the message that we're all friendly and informal and welcoming, but I still think it's questionable practice. It can be quite insulting. I know that my parents would never dream of calling the lady next door by her first name, and they've known her over 30 years. I also think that sharing rooms is simply not acceptable. Would you want to share a room permanently with a stranger, or a succession of strangers, who may be suffering from all kinds of illnesses? (Residential care worker)*

In a press release issued in November 1998, Frank Dobson, Secretary of State for Health, announced a programme to establish standards of NHS care for older people:

> *We have made a start on dealing with the privacy and dignity concerns [about older people] and gender discrimination. ... Existing plans for new mixed sex wards were abandoned and the NHS is now embarked on a major drive to eliminate mixed sex wards. By 2002 we will have cut the number of mixed sex wards from one in three to just one in twenty. (Department of Health, 1998)*

Activity

Follow these instructions then get a colleague to critically reflect on your communication skills and the knowledge you have assimilated from your patient during this interaction.

Take a position near the older person. You should be close enough to be able to reach out and touch them, if desired. The most comfortable arrangement is to have the chairs at 45° to each other. If possible, the chairs should be the same height and you should not stand or walk during the conversation. Your patient may have a hearing problem or may not understand your accent. Remember clarity of speech and the use of simple sentences are most effective in communicating with older people. Engage in effective communication skills that will elicit significant information from your patient so you can make a clinical assessment.

Active and systematic inquiry

A health-care professional should inquire about the common physical symptoms of later life (such as visual and hearing defects, falls and weight loss) and typical psychosocial events (death of a loved one, change in living arrangements, recent retirement, financial setback, feelings of decreased self-esteem, hopelessness and anxiety) as this type of inquiry demonstrates a personal interest and may uncover unreported maladies.

Interview pacing

Older people should be given sufficient time to respond to your questions. As a rule, older people do not find silences as uncomfortable as they might seem to you. In fact, this silence frequently gives them an opportunity to formulate answers to questions, and to elaborate on certain points. Not only can a slow and relaxed pace in the interview decrease their anxiety, it can also provide you with much more information to use.

Non-verbal clues

Be continually alert for changes in facial expression, gestures, postures and touch as additional methods of communication during a conversation with an older person. These non-verbal signs can provide considerable information about conditions such as depression or anxiety.

Comfort and calming

Touch may also be an effective way to relax the conversational atmosphere and make contact with an older person. An older person may be less inhibited about physical touch from a caregiver. Holding your patient's hand or resting your hand on a patient's arm may be very reassuring when dealing with potentially stressful or emotional matters during an interview.

Optimistic realism

It can be easy for health-care professionals working with older persons to try to deny the problems of later life, but neither you nor your patient believes phrases like 'you'll live to be 120' or 'it's nothing to worry about'. Avoid using them. Yet don't abandon all hope for an older patient and concentrate your efforts on what should work in the here and now.

CONDITIONS THAT CREATE COMMUNICATIONS CHALLENGES

Despite major advances in the ability to prolong life, a significant level of illness and disability – stroke, dementia, hearing loss and visual problems – often comes with increased age. The most prevalent of age-related disabilities are those involving communication (Jacobs-Condit, 1984). In the US there are more than 8 million older adults with communication difficulties, the majority of whom are hearing-impaired, whereas in the UK at least 60% of people over 70 (living at home and in care) are affected by hearing impairment (Macphee *et al.*, 1998).

Although the overall incidence of visual impairment in the UK is unknown, the Royal College of Ophthalmologists has reported an increase in the occurrence of cataracts, glaucoma and degeneration of the retina in people aged over 65. It is thought that numbers of people registering for blindness and partial sight underestimate the problem by over 50% (Office of Population Censuses and Surveys, 1999). Communication is affected by visual problems since it is more difficult to share information if someone is unable to observe body language, see what you are referring to, watch television or recognize people.

Depression

Clinical depression is a common psychological change following the onset of dysphasia, as described in this extract from *Dysphasia Matters: A Medical Teaching Pack* (Action for Dysphasic Adults, 1997):

> *Doctors should actively look for signs of depression in dysphasic patients to avoid leaving it untreated, as the dysphasic patient may not be able to describe their mood and other symptoms. Depression may begin during the first weeks after the onset of dysphasia but often starts months or even years later in response to the many lifestyle changes which occur with dysphasia. A depressed patient is likely to make slower progress in rehabilitation and have a poorer outcome.*

To learn more about the emotional effects of communication problems, you may like to read *The Impact of Language Loss on Marriage* (Sparkes, 1993) and *Assessment and Management of Emotional and Psychosocial Reactions to Brain Damage and Aphasia* (Wahrborg, 1991).

Expressive impairment

Speech impairments are also common in older people. Nearly 75% of all strokes occur in people aged 65 or over and nearly 60% of those who survive strokes experience speech and language difficulties. Reading and writing may also be affected, and so may non-verbal communication such as facial expression, voice tone and emphasis.

Dysphasia

People affected by dysphasia often experience feelings of isolation and of not being part of a group or the wider community: 'Dysphasia usually has far-reaching effects on a person's ability to access and maintain social networks and participate in community life. This is not surprising since most social interaction involves verbal communication' (Action for Dysphasic Adults, 1997). Dysphasia is a language impairment affecting people's ability to express themselves and understand another's language. They may have difficulty

- choosing the right word;
- putting the right speech sounds into the word;
- correcting speech errors;
- arranging words into sentences;
- understanding long or complex sentences;
- reading;
- spelling.

Dysphasia can be so severe that the sufferer is unable to make themselves understood, or so mild that only the dysphasic person is aware of it. It can affect people of any age, and often occurs in stroke patients. Here are some dos and don'ts adapted from Gravell (1988).

Dos
- Do talk in a quiet, relaxed atmosphere free from distractions.
- Do gain the person's attention before speaking, perhaps by touching the person or saying his or her name.
- Do use facial expressions and gestures to back up your words.
- Do speak somewhat more slowly than usual; keep your utterances short, simple and direct but not childlike. Emphasize key words but don't raise your voice.
- Do be prepared to repeat more than usual, but don't try to get through by volume.
- Do ask simple, direct questions.
- Do ask questions to clarify what the person wants to say. Dysphasic people may have difficulty in selecting the word they want and in knowing when this is occurring.
- Do ask closed questions, questions for which the individual could answer with yes, no or with a fact.
- Do remember that the person's ability may fluctuate; being able to say a word one day does not mean they will be able to say it the next day.
- Do encourage all attempts to communicate, whether by word, facial expression or gesture.

Don'ts
- Don't be surprised if the dysphasic person swears; their swearing may upset them too.
- Don't correct the person's errors.
- Don't pressurize the person to respond.
- Don't discuss vague, abstract topics.
- Don't talk for the person; you may put words into his or her mouth.
- Don't discuss the person in his or her presence.

Dysphasia does not imply mental handicap. Dysphasic people are usually competent to make their own decisions if information is presented in a way that enables them to be informed and to understand and if they are helped to communicate their wishes and decisions.

Dysarthria

Dysarthria is a speech impairment affecting the person's ability to achieve precise movements of the larynx, palate, tongue or lips. It may have several effects:

- slurred speech sounds
- nasal speech
- a quiet voice

- slow rate of speech
- speech sounds omitted.

At worst, the person may be unintelligible. People with dysarthria are sometimes wrongly thought to have drunk too much alcohol. Here are some dos and don'ts adapted from Gravell (1988).

Dos
- Do be patient and tolerant, as their speech will be slow and take great effort. Remind them that you will give them time to get their message across.
- Do make the surroundings quiet.
- Do face the speaker so you can watch their mouth and facial movements.
- Do provide paper and pencil if the person is physically able to write or draw.
- Do provide pictures or other recommended aids to supplement speech or take the place of speech.
- Do encourage speech efforts.
- Do repeat the parts of the message you can understand, so that the speaker does not have to go through those parts again.
- Do ask appropriate questions to establish clearly what is meant.
- Do ask for a message to be repeated if necessary; perhaps ask for one word at a time or for a particular word to be spelled out.
- Do let the speaker know the optimal rate of speech that you can understand.
- Do seek specific advice from the speech and language therapist.

Don'ts
- Don't pretend that you've understood something if you haven't.
- Don't demand lengthy, complex responses as this will tire the patient.
- Don't persist when the person is tired; try again after the person has rested.
- Don't speak at the same time as the person and don't interrupt.
- Don't raise your voice unless the person has a hearing problem.

Neurological and physical difficulties

With age, the physical systems of the body become more vulnerable to progressive neurological difficulties. Parkinson's disease, the most common age-related disease of the basal ganglia, affects about 1 in 100 people over age 60 (and roughly 25% of people over 85) and is associated with motor speech control problems. A range of voice problems, such as inadequate loudness and a disabling variation in speech quality, constitute 22% of the communication difficulties seen in nursing home patients. Figure 6.3 shows a health-care team encouraging a patient to maintain mobility.

Other expressive communication problems may occur in people with

Figure 6.3

Maintaining physical mobility

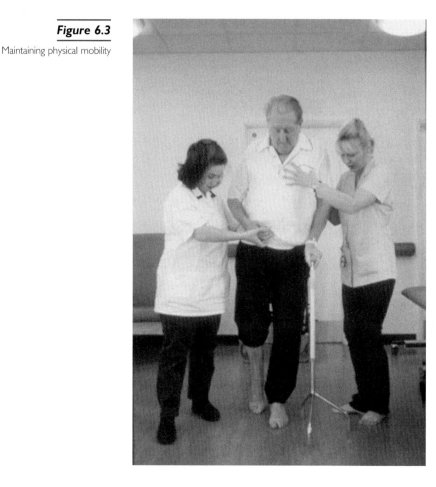

head and neck cancer who have undergone major surgery to remove tumours, for example, partial or total glossectomy or laryngectomy. They often require communication support, including technological interventions such as changing and refitting speech valves. Speech can be achieved, with help, through a servox, which vibrates under the chin to achieve an electronic-sounding voice, or a post-surgical voice prosthesis.

Alzheimer's disease and other dementias

Alzheimer's disease affects around 15–20% of the population over age 65. Language disturbance is symptomatic of dementia, often occurring at an early stage. Dementia care is probably the most challenging of all work with older people. It makes great demands on relatives and care staff. It can offer no hope of cure. Many societies, including our own, are prone to categorizing older people as incompetent, ugly and burdensome. Older people who have dementia are often subjected to ageism in its most extreme form. They are virtually dehumanized and perceived as not real persons.

According to Griffiths (1991), language breakdown during dementia occurs in these broad stages:

- Speech becomes empty and vague; sentences are not completed.
- Word finding becomes a problem; the person has increasing difficulty naming things.
- Speech becomes increasingly repetitive.
- Speech and conversation are related only to the individual.
- Mutism may follow.

This inability to communicate can irritate and sometimes overwhelm staff. Confronting dementia causes much trepidation, not least among nurses, other health-care workers and other professionals.

Tom Kitson was a pioneer in articulating the social construction of dementia. He challenged the dominance of biomedical explanations for the disease. In his book *Dementia Reconsidered* (Kitson, 1997) he identifies two kinds of anxiety:

> *First, naturally enough, every human being is afraid of becoming frail and highly dependent, fears which are amplified in any society where the sense of community is weak or missing. Added to that, there is the fear of a long, drawn-out process of dying and of death itself. Contact with those who are elderly, weak and vulnerable activates these fears and threatens our basic sense of security. Second, we all carry fears about mental instability. The thought of being lost forever in confusion is terrifying. Many people have come close to this at some point, for example at a time of great stress. When we witness dementia in another person we can feel both kinds of fear: fear of dependence and frailty, and fear of going insane. There is no real consolation in saying: 'It will never happen to me,' as we can do with many other anxiety-provoking conditions. Dementia is present in almost every street, and discussed repeatedly in the media. People from all kinds of background are affected, so in being close to a person with dementia we may be seeing some terrifying anticipation of how we might become.*

Kitson suggests that it is not surprising if we resort to the defensive tactic of 'turning those who have dementia into a different species, not persons in the full sense'. He then identifies the principal problem as being 'not that of changing people with dementia, or of "managing" their behaviour; it is that of moving beyond our own anxieties and defences, so that true meeting can occur, and life-giving relationships can grow'.

Personhood

Kitson's (1997) approach, and the approaches of other practitioners working with people experiencing dementia, is based on the principle of 'personhood'. This 'acknowledges the unique subjectivity of the person with dementia – their unique way of experiencing life and relationships' and seeks to validate that experience and the reality of their feelings. Earlier approaches to dementia care tended to regard the behaviour of the person as meaningless. However, by establishing and maintaining the concept of personhood, the meaning of behaviour that may seem irrational and problematic can be uncovered. The essence of this principle is appropriate and effective communication.

There is a growing body of research describing the effectiveness of these psychosocial methods. It is now widely acknowledged that challenging behaviours on the part of patients with dementia may not always be a result of brain damage alone; they may instead be an attempt to communicate basic human needs. Here are some dos and don'ts.

Dos
- Do make sure aids such as hearing aids and glasses are worn if appropriate.
- Do display pictures of family and friends and any people with whom the individual has frequent contact.
- Do establish a simple, consistent routine and environment.
- Do make sure you are calm and have a relaxed facial expression and posture.
- Do minimize distractions such as television, radio and other people chattering or working in the room; if necessary, take the person to a quiet place.
- Do gain the person's attention before speaking to them.
- Do speak simply and slowly. Use short sentences, ideally having around seven words. Introduce only one idea per sentence.
- Do use frequent reminders of time, place and person such as the person's name and daily events. You could say, 'It's four o'clock, time for tea, Elisabeth.'
- Do allow the person time to answer. Someone with moderate dementia takes five times as long to process information as an older person without dementia.
- Do listen actively. Learn to pick up cues and prompts.
- Do listen for the meaning behind the words. People with dementia often use metaphors to communicate.
- Do check that you've understood what's been said. You could say, 'So you want a cup of tea, Elisabeth?'
- Do be prepared for a display of emotion. Many people are grateful for the opportunity to communicate.
- Do be tactful when returning to a topic if the conversation seems rambling or odd.
- Do use touch and gestures to reinforce your presence and what you are saying.
- Do mean what you say. Because they have difficulty processing verbal communication, people with dementia appear to be very sensitive to body language.
- Do use open postures, sit at the same level and make eye contact.

- Do encourage any attempts to communicate. Let the person know that you realize the effort they have made to communicate and show that you appreciate it.
- Do allow the person to talk about the 'old days'. Link this with the present to orient the person to reality. You could say, 'Margot had light hair when she was young. Now her hair is dark.'

Don'ts

- Don't force the person to carry on if you feel the conversation is going nowhere.
- Don't avoid communication because you feel it may upset the person. You are actually helping and enabling the person to express their thoughts and feelings.
- Don't argue or try to solve a disagreement; change the subject instead.
- Don't be sarcastic.
- Don't laugh at their attempts to communicate with you. They are trying very hard. Never denigrate their efforts or strip them of their dignity.
- Don't use anecdotes or complex explanations.
- Don't appear rushed, even if you are.
- Don't speak to the person as though they were a child.
- Don't be confusing. Don't twiddle your earrings while discussing teeth.
- Don't assume that lack of response means lack of understanding. The person may be thinking or may not wish to respond.
- Don't reward inappropriate language, but don't give up if thought processes or words get mixed up. You may still be able to understand what is being said.

Differences between dementia and dysphasia

Table 6.1 shows the main differences between dementia and dysphasia. Consider how older people with dementia spend their days and think about their restricted view of the world. Here are some ways they may spend their time:

- sitting in the same place, in the same chair
- feeling the textures of cotton, polyester cotton or nylon

Dysphasia	Dementia
Sudden onset	Gradual onset
Stable or improving	Deteriorating
Focal lesion	Diffuse brain damage
Intellect preserved	Intellect impaired
Communicative functions impaired	Global impairment
Sensory integration therapy	

Table 6.1

The main differences between dementia and dysphasia

- hearing blaring television sets or the noise and bustle of other people and staff
- smelling mainly air freshener, furniture polish and soap
- being touched only when care is required
- being cared for in a constant temperature
- having no idea of the weather or of the passing of the seasons
- rarely getting the opportunity to go out.

Routine is important to people with dementia. It helps them to make sense of their world and their lives. Nonetheless, you may wish to investigate and introduce sensory integration therapy into your care of patients with dementia. Find out about it from the Association of Occupational Therapists. Insights and practical advice on all aspects of Alzheimer's disease and other forms of dementia can be found at www.alzheimers.org.uk, the website of the Alzheimer's Disease Society.

TECHNOLOGY AIDS COMMUNICATION

Caring for older people often involves becoming familiar with assistive technologies. Assistive technologies can contribute to the care and comfort of older people in institutional settings as well as at home. As each individual is different, you should do a proper needs assessment to determine what technology may be appropriate and to provide sufficient orientation so the new devices are correctly incorporated into the patient's lifestyle. Devices frequently allow older people to remain longer in their own homes and to communicate more readily with those around them. Some assistive technologies are low-tech and rather inexpensive, whereas others are high-tech and quite costly.

The effect of drugs on speech

Pharmaceuticals affect an older person's communication abilities. Although many drugs are known to alter the articulation of speech, there has been little systematic research on these effects, particularly among older people. Alcohol is probably the most readily recognized speech-affecting drug, but numerous prescribed medications can significantly influence articulation, sequencing and speech patterns. Commonly prescribed drugs such as the benzodiazepine derivatives can, in large doses, cause slurring of speech, but even therapeutic doses affect higher functions of speech. They can cause the individual to use greater numbers of words, make unintelligible or inaudible remarks, or be unable to complete sentences. Anticonvulsants such as phenobarbitone have a marked effect on cerebellar functions, and therefore speech, when their levels are too high. Individuals with Parkinson's disease treated with levodopa often show an initial increase in speech intelligibility, although this benefit can be short-lived due to other side effects of the drug (Garwel, 1981).

Low-technology interventions

Alongside the deployment of increasingly complex technology, there are always opportunities to help older people communicate effectively using less sophisticated aids. Depending on the nature of the communication difficulty, various creative and often simple tactics can be used by enterprising nurses, carers and therapists. Here are some examples:

- Use picture boards.
- Show the patient items such as tea or coffee jars and watch for the direction of their eyes.
- Provide illustrated menus to help patients select their food.
- Together, you and the patient compile a personalized word book of everyday vocabulary. This is a notebook or word diary comprising words that you both agree are relevant to the patient's needs and experiences. Some entries could be the names of people in the patient's family.
- Devise a personalized system of gestures where you and the patient agree on their meaning and usefulness. For example, you may devise a gesture to illustrate a family member who wears glasses or who is very tall.
- Supply pen and paper on which the patient can write or draw messages.
- Provide an interpreter for a patient whose mother tongue is not English.
- Provide an interpreter who can understand a patient with expressive impairments.
- Reduce ambient noise such as the sound of the television or radio.
- Reduce visual and other distractions, and ensure good lighting.
- If the patient has a hearing aid or glasses, check that they are working and that the patient is wearing them.
- Ensure the patient is physically comfortable, otherwise they will find it difficult to concentrate.

Use your patient's name. Develop eye contact. Listen and observe. To find out how best to help a patient communicate, ask the patient what helps and consult a speech and language therapist.

Activity

Refer to and work with the speech and language therapist to obtain as much information as possible about the communication abilities of your older patients. Ask what you can do to help. Watch for signs of improvement in communication, including your patient's ability to write and draw.

Hearing impairment and aids for hearing

Try to recognize hearing impairment in older people. Once recognized, it can be treated effectively with a modern hearing aid. Previously it was thought that investigation by pure tone audiometry was the only reliable method of detecting hearing loss in older people, but this puts considerable pressure on qualified staff. There are simply not enough local audiology and otolaryngology services to cope with the increasing numbers of older people who would benefit from testing and subsequent treatment.

You can help to save time and anguish for those with a hearing impairment by remembering two simple points:

- Wax in people's ears affects hearing. It is simple and easy to treat; clinics will not usually test hearing unless the person's ears are free of wax.
- The patient may have tonal loss. High pitch is lost first, so people with a hearing impairment usually find men easier to hear than women. You could lower your voice an octave to facilitate communication.

One study discovered a cheap, available and decidedly low-tech strategy that has achieved a consistently high success rate in detecting hearing impairment in older patients: 'We recommend referral to a specialist of those patients who fail to hear a whispered voice at 2 feet and who would accept provision of an aid' (Macphee *et al.*, 1988). And here is someone's response to their mother's dementia:

> *My mother's dementia bewilders and isolates her and, sadly, her family and friends have had to resign themselves to this. What we cannot accept, however, is the added isolation of her deafness. Yes, she used to cope with her hearing aid, albeit with difficulty. In her present condition, remembering where it is and then what to do with it is quite beyond her and she has given up the struggle. How can you expect elderly people, many of whom have failing eyesight and less than fine motor skills, to twiddle miniature wheels and tiny buttons? I shall scour the antique shops for an old-fashioned ear trumpet. Small may be cosmetically beautiful but large and manageably simple would suit us. I want to chat with my mother, not shout at her.*

Individuals with hearing impairments can benefit from a simple blinking light instead of a doorbell and with clocks that have a flashing light alarm. Other devices incorporate an electronic voice, such as speaking calendars and speaking clocks.

High-technology interventions

Technology will inevitably play an increased role in the assessment and management of communication impairment. Many aids are already in use:

- listening devices and other sensory aids for auditory and visual impairments
- prosthetic speech aids

- instruments for assessing speech, language and auditory functions
- computer and telecommunications-based electronic treatment programmes.

Many people think that electronic aids, such as that used by Professor Stephen Hawking, are the answer for those who are unable to speak. However, this type of technology is still insignificant for most older people. Electronic communication aids, although simple in comparison with personal computers, are expensive and not widely used by the majority of older people in conversational settings. The most commonly used devices are hearing aids and adapted telephones, for example textphones.

Perhaps it is only possible to understand what is involved in using communication aids if you try to rely on one in a real, conversational setting:

> *Auntie Adrian, living in Kenya, suffered from the increasingly debilitating effects of motor neurone disease which was diagnosed when she was 73 years old. By 85, she could no longer speak. She expressed herself with the help of a keyboard and a two-way screen, which we could read when sitting opposite it, and which she could read as well. Adrian could not manipulate her arms, hands or fingers to use the keyboard. So her domestic aide, a man aged 35 who had known Adrian since he was eight years old, gently and sensitively held her right arm. He was the only person able to sense her tiniest movement toward the letters of her keyboard when she wished to spell out her thoughts and greetings. We would respond verbally, and together Adrian and her helper would slowly tap the keyboard so that we could read her response again on the screen. It was intensely slow, but it worked.*

Electronic monitoring

Several forms of electronic monitoring are becoming increasingly available for older people. One form is video monitoring or closed-circuit television and another form involves motion sensors. Video monitoring involves placing a camera in the patient's location with a monitor at a remote location. Transmission of signals can take place using a telephone line; access to the system requires personal identification numbers, giving high privacy (Miskelly, 2001). These devices may be found in institutional settings as well as home care. Motion sensors have been incorporated in fall detectors. These monitors can transmit information about a person falling so that an alarm is set off locally or at a remote location. Some of these devices use telephone lines and some are wireless.

EFFECTIVE COMMUNICATION WITHIN THE CARING TEAM

Effective communication with carers is as important as it is with patients. 'The NHS ignores the six million carers who support members of their family at home,' says a survey conducted by the Carers National Association (Henwood, 1998). Henwood found that although carers are one of the health service's most valuable assets, NHS staff are unaware of their needs and fail to support them by providing help and information. According to this report, 1 in 3 carers said that their concerns had been ignored when discharge was being organized and only 14% of those discharged had been visited by their GP to see if they were managing.

Caring for a person with dementia at home saves the state an average of £20 688 per year in nursing home costs (Holmes *et al.*, 1998). Many carers are surprised to discover how difficult it is to gain access to services that will allow them to care for their family members at home. They may even feel that they are asking too much. Some health-care practitioners assume that the person being cared for is a burden to the carer. However, many carers feel fulfilled in that role, especially if they receive sufficient and regular support.

Working together

The NMC recognizes the complexity of health care and stresses the need to appreciate the contribution of professional health-care staff, students, supporting staff and also voluntary and independent agencies. The provision of care is now a multiprofessional, multi-agency activity and to work effectively it must be based on mutual understanding, trust, respect and cooperation. Patients and clients are equal partners with health professionals in their care, and therefore they have the right to be involved in decisions about their care. It is clearly impossible for any one profession to possess all the knowledge, skills and resources needed to meet the total health-care needs of society. Good care will be the product of a good team. All members of the team are entitled to equality and each member must not be discriminated against because of gender, age, race, disability, sexuality, culture or religious beliefs. There needs to be effective communication and teamwork to make sure these principles are not neglected.

Many organizations, including charities, provide support for carers. Increasingly, these organizations use websites to provide carers and patients with helpful information. Many relatives of older people may be carers. A carer is someone who takes responsibility for the everyday living tasks and/or emotional well-being of a disabled, frail or ill relative, partner or friend.

Establishing and maintaining good communication with relatives, who may also be older and vulnerable themselves, is an important factor in the patient's well-being. When an older person dies, they leave behind a web of friends and relatives who may themselves be in need of support. Where possible, community and district nurses need to establish and maintain contact with the former patient's spouse, relatives, carer and close friends following his or her death. This contact could have a positive impact on the quality of life of older people. Here is what McCormack (1997) has to say:

Many older people feel socially isolated, and one of the multitude of unfortunate side-effects of social isolation is that it can lead to malnutrition in older people living alone. When an older person loses a spouse, sibling or friend, social networks begin to deteriorate, and lack of socialisation associated with food – a meal out, a pint and a sandwich in the pub, visiting a friend for tea and a chat – leads to a marked reduction in eating. People who live alone, men in particular, are reported to have a lower nutritional intake than those who live with their spouse or some other person. When the companionship and social support of a spouse during shopping, meal preparation and eating together is no longer there, depression can set in. And a major feature of depression is loss of appetite.

And here is an example from Forster (1989):

No family could be more devoted. Mum goes at two o'clock and stays until four when I arrive and I stay until five when Adrian arrives and Adrian either leaves at half past or stays a little later if dad isn't going to be able to get there until seven.

Cultural issues

When considering communication with people whose cultures are different from our own, we may wonder whether we all speak the same language. Although a shared language is a major factor in communicating, something else is equally important – culturally specific behaviour. Understanding the cultural norms and behaviour of those from different backgrounds helps us to communicate. Age Concern England (www.ace.org.uk) supported the establishment of the Black and Minority Ethnic Elders Forum in 2002 with the goal to achieve tangible change and real improvements to the lives of black and minority ethnic elders in England. Minority ethnic groups are the fastest-ageing groups within the population. By 2030 it is projected that the minority ethnic elder population will have increased tenfold from 175 000 to 1.7 million, yet many suffer poor health, live in inadequate housing and experience low incomes even more commonly than other pensioners. So how do we develop an understanding? Where do we start? The term 'culture' is commonly used to denote shared ways of behaving in recognisable groups. Shared behaviour embraces many things, including non-verbal communication as well as verbal communication.

Non-verbal communication

Non-verbal communication is powerful and eloquent. If we understand the non-verbal communication of another person, we can usually communicate effectively without words. If we do not understand and therefore misinterpret the other person's body posture, gestures, facial expressions, and so on, we will not communicate effectively. Consider the views of this nurse teacher:

In my early years as a nurse teacher, I had very little contact with people from cultures other than my own. When I later worked with a student who was from another culture, I found that her hand-washing left a lot to be desired, and I sat down with her to discuss the problem. The more I pointed out the risks to patients from poor attention to hand hygiene, the more broadly she smiled. I became annoyed and in the end said that I didn't think risking spreading infection was anything to smile about. A few years later I started studying cultural issues in depth and found to my horror that in that student's culture, smiling is a polite way of showing acceptance of criticism – the stronger the 'offence', the broader the smile.

It is important to understand the non-verbal communication of people from other cultures. To get started, you could carry out a literature search, although this may not yield the detail you need about a particular culture. A more direct way is to ask people who belong to those cultures. Ask people who speak your language and who understand your culture well enough to point out the major differences between their culture and yours. For some Asian people, making eye contact on first meeting is considered offensive. This is just one example of how you need to consider the cultural background of your patients. Bear in mind that we ourselves may be members of minority ethnic or cultural groups in certain situations, for example, a German working in Wales, an Afro-Caribbean working in Scotland, a Canadian working in England.

Verbal communication

Verbal communication requires shared language. Some older people may have coped well enough using their second language when they were younger, but may have reverted to their first language when they became more frail, confused and generally more vulnerable. Others may have lived in an alien culture for several decades without learning the language of that culture:

Elsie is an example of an old immigrant woman who is growing old in an institution. Elsie knows three words of English although she spends 80% of her time in a hospital geriatric ward. I cannot present a quote from Elsie because I do not speak Italian. What I can say about Elsie is what I have heard from the nursing staff. She talks to herself (not that she has anyone else to talk to on the ward). She hallucinates and she is delusional. I do not know how they have drawn these conclusions, given that none of them speak Italian, either. (Skodra, 1992)

There are several ways of attempting to overcome the lack of a shared language between patient and health-care professional, some more effective and accessible than others. In areas where there are relatively large groups of minorities who do not speak English, health providers may employ link workers from those groups. These link workers not only understand the cultural norms and language of the group, but are also trained in medical and nursing interpretation. If, for example, they are asked by nurses to help them explore the reasons why an older woman from a particular Asian culture is constipated, they will be able to converse with the patient in her own language using appropriate translations relating to the problem. The link worker will understand that it may be essential to communicate where males who are not close family members cannot overhear the conversation. The link worker will also be able to help nursing staff provide culturally appropriate circumstances for the woman to open her bowels: the opportunity to wash her genital and anal area with running water after using the lavatory, without which her culture dictates that she simply will not open her bowels.

The *Black and Ethnic Minority Groups in England: Health and Lifestyles* (Rudat, 1994) surveyed Caribbean, Indian, Pakistani and Bangladeshi ethnic groups. It gave an indication of the considerable need for link workers, advocates and interpreters and of their relatively poor provision. Where link workers are not available it may still be possible to use an interpreting service, either face-to-face or by telephone. Failing that, drawing and sign language can achieve a great deal in an emergency.

Activity

Reflect on issues that could emerge if a family member is used as an interpreter. For example, it may not be appropriate to communicate a mother's intimate medical details to her son, or a parent's poor prognosis to a young daughter or son. It may be better to seek out local interpreters with professional experience of interpretation who understand and respect the need for confidentiality. However, this too may not be suitable for every patient. If you plan to use an interpreter, make certain that the patient and the carers are happy with the person selected. If they are not happy, then seek someone else or seek a different method.

If you are interested in learning more about working with patients from other cultures and about advocacy in this context, you might like to contact Age Concern (www.ageconcern.org.uk) about their conference On Your Side, which took place in September 1999 as well as further work to date.

Counselling

Perkins and Poynton (1990) investigated the effects of providing group counselling for relatives of hospitalized dementia patients. There were three significant findings:

- Probably the most important finding was that group counselling significantly increased the morale and well-being of relatives. This increase was not only apparent immediately after the group sessions, but was maintained three months later.

● The relatives gained more knowledge about the nature and course of dementia. Interestingly, virtually all the relatives had already received accurate guidance and literature from an Alzheimer's disease support organization. This suggests that it is not the information alone that the relatives needed, but the supportive environment of the group to be able fully to assimilate and accept the real nature and course of the dementia process.

● The relatives showed a significant change in their behaviour when they visited the patient. They had a much greater repertoire of psychosocial and physical activities with the patient, for example, reading newspapers, looking at family photographs, playing music, dancing, singing, and playing games. The relatives said that engaging in such activities helped to reduce the helplessness and distress they experienced during visiting periods because they elicited responses from the patient.

Make contact with a regional dementia centre. Your local library can give you contact details and a number of websites provide helpful information. Effective communication between health workers, care workers, the patient and relatives can lead to successful, integrated health care.

Services for older people provide a challenging context for developing communication and information systems. In the past, agencies have concentrated efforts on internal communications and information systems used within agencies. Due to the wide range of services that support older people, it has been difficult to produce comprehensive information systems that can talk to each other across different agencies. In the absence of fully integrated computer information systems, good human communication among workers from different agencies becomes critical.

As the number of frail older adults requiring care and treatment rises, effective communication between groups of professionals becomes essential. Hospital, nursing home and community practitioners, including physiotherapists, speech and language therapists and dieticians, must liaise and exchange pertinent information.

Community and primary care

Consider this extract from Langlands and Moores (1999):

Nurses, midwives and health visitors working in primary and community care are developing their roles to help provide modern and dependable services. They act as health promoters, giving information to patients, assessing health issues and screening for early signs of treatable disease. They are public health workers, focusing on whole communities as well as individuals, fulfilling the public health functions of community profiling, health needs assessment, communicable disease control and community development. Health

> *visitors and community nurses, working close to where people live in local communities are acting as advocates for vulnerable groups and people who are socially excluded, making sure they have access to mainstream health services.*

The following example of effective communication (Flaxman, 1997) promotes seamless care between sectors. One hospital trust investigated how it could reduce the seemingly inevitable winter acute admission crisis by involving general practice at an early stage and taking preventive measures in a larger and more targeted way. High-risk patients were identified and allocated to a specific practice or district nurse, who visited them in late October. Their needs were noted and acted upon where necessary, mainly flu immunization and checking the status of any other relevant conditions, such as asthma and bronchitis. The patients were then advised to contact their specified nurse directly at the onset of any flu-like or relevant symptoms, so that they could be treated immediately. Other health-care professionals such as physiotherapists, occupational therapists and social workers were involved or made aware of the patients' needs from the outset.

Not only was this experiment in interprofessional communication and coordination of care successful in preventing a considerable amount of needless suffering for the at-risk older person, it also saved money. The general practice involved estimated that the project would be self-financing if it prevented 12 emergency admissions, a total that was comfortably exceeded.

IMPORTANCE OF FULL AND ACCURATE RECORDS

The documentation that health professionals keep about their patients serves several purposes. First and foremost, records should delineate what has been done so that others can understand the needs, treatments and responses to treatments; it is a written form of communication. All documentation should meet professional standards as described in NMC guidelines (NMC, 2002b). These records can also be produced as legal documents before a court of law and/or by

- the health service commissioner;
- the NMC in relation to a professional conduct committee hearing; or
- managers at a local level to facilitate an inquiry or investigation.

There are several important principles for keeping good records. First, there is what goes into a record and how the records look. Then there are some legal issues that you should consider in your own record-keeping practice. Although the standards may vary among different health-care professionals and in different work settings, all records should be created in a systematic and logical manner.

Clear and complete records

The NMC has identified a number of factors that contribute to effective record-keeping:

- Records should be factual, consistent and accurate.
- Records should be written as soon as possible after an event has occurred, providing current information on the care and condition of the patient or client.
- Records should be written clearly and so the text cannot be erased.
- Records should be written so that any alterations or additions are dated, timed and signed and so the original entry can still be read clearly.
- Records should be accurately dated, timed and signed with the signature printed alongside the first entry.
- Records should not include abbreviations, jargon, meaningless phrases, irrelevant speculation and offensive subjective statements.
- Records should be readable on any photocopies.

Here are some other things to consider (NMC, 2002b):

- Records should be written, wherever possible, with the involvement of the patient, the client or their carer.
- Records should be written in terms that the patient or client can understand.
- Records should be consecutive.
- Records should identify problems that have arisen and the action taken to rectify them.
- Records should provide clear evidence of the care planned, the decisions made, the care delivered and the information shared.

Legal implications

As a health-care professional, you have a professional duty of care and a legal duty of care. Therefore, according to NMC (2002b), your record-keeping needs to demonstrate

- a full account of your assessment and the care you have planned and provided;
- relevant information about the condition of the patient or client at any given time;
- measures you have taken to respond to a patient's needs;
- evidence that you have understood and honoured your duty of care, that you have taken all reasonable steps to care for the patient or client and that any actions or omissions on your part have not compromised their safety in any way;
- a record of any arrangements you have made for the continuing care of a patient or client.

Other members of the health-care team can assist you in understanding what needs to be recorded and how often entries are made, as circumstances can vary from patient to patient and from setting to setting. However, courts of law tend to take the view that 'if it is not recorded, it has not been done'. Thus, you will find that you will frequently have to use your professional judgement to decide what is relevant and what should be recorded. On some occasions you may be working with older persons who are subject to mental health legislation and you must ensure that you have a thorough working knowledge of how these laws apply to your particular area of practice. When making entries in records for these clients, you must comply as appropriate with the guidance given by the Mental Health Act Commission for England and Wales, the Mental Welfare Commission for Scotland or the Mental Health Commission for Northern Ireland. When making any record, always remember that other members of the health-care team are relying on your records. Clear, accurate and complete communication is always essential.

An increasing number of health-care professionals regularly use information technology to record the planning, assessment and delivery of care. There are many advantages to computerized records as generally they are easier to read, they are less bulky, they reduce the need for duplication and they can increase communication across the interprofessional health-care team. All the basic principles that apply to manual records also apply to computerized records. In particular, the principles about confidentiality must be preserved to ensure that records are secure and that information shared electronically is held in strict confidence. In the end, even though computerized records increase communication of important information with others on the team, there is still a need to maintain ongoing dialogue.

Consequently, it is important that records are clear, accurate, comprehensive and informative. For example, James has quite clearly sustained an injury that he might otherwise not have sustained, or which would have been discovered earlier if action had been taken at the appropriate time and if other carers had been made aware of the situation. The nurse in this case does not appear to have made or maintained any documentation about the individual incident (accident report) or about the assessment and actions taken in relation to finding James. This contravenes the Code of Professional Conduct (NMC, 2002a) and is also dangerous practice for the nurse, not least because the legal precedent that is usually followed is 'if it is not written down, it was not done' (NMC, 2002b). The nurse in this case will have to explain his actions and the consequences, but with no documentation to help. Having a written document does not prove that the care was given, but it does demonstrate the intention to provide care and to take action. Besides the uses described above, documents written by nurses can be used as part of an audit, quality control or inspection process.

Words

When writing documents, health-care professionals are often faced with the problem of knowing what to write and how to write it. Sometimes we literally cannot remember a word or, more often, we try to use words we do not fully understand, but think might be right. Consider this anecdote:

> *While visiting my mum in a nursing home one evening, I overheard two nurses asking, while writing up patient records: 'What's that word for patients passing a lot of urine at night? Is it "nocturia"? Let's look it up in the dictionary.' I thought, if they have to look it up, the other nurses probably won't understand it either.*

A simple remedy to this situation is the right rule. Avoid using a word unless you are comfortable with it and know that it's the right word. Then use the right word at the right time for the right thing. Be concise and direct, say what you mean and mean what you say. Avoid ambiguous words and phrases.

Record-keeping and seamless care

The NMC states that registered nurses must demonstrate their accountability for the entries made by others who are not trained but are under their supervision, such as health-care assistants or pre-registration students of nursing, by countersigning their entries (NMC, 2002a). However, the NMC has received many letters from nurses explaining the difficulties of doing this, pointing out that there are not enough nurses and complaining that older people with nursing needs are often placed in residential homes (NMC, 2002a).

Multidisciplinary record-keeping

D'Sa (1995) described the introduction of a multidisciplinary system of record-keeping to a ward caring for elderly persons. All members of the multidisciplinary team were encouraged to contribute to 'progress notes'. Evaluation by the ward staff indicated that communication between the team members had been enhanced and care planning and goal-setting have been improved. Storing all records in a single folder made it easier to find patient information. Staff found the introduction of multidisciplinary notes was a good thing. They said there was less repetition and better communication between disciplines. The reduction in entries suggested that staff spent less time writing notes and more time with patients.

Activity————————————————————

Identify the people involved in caring for Mary. Now do the following steps:
- On a five-point scale from exemplary to satisfactory, note the quality of service that Mary received from each of her carers.
- For each unsatisfactory mark, note what action would have made communication more effective.

- Make notes on any repercussions each action would have on health and care service colleagues, Mary's relatives, Mary herself, and others.
- Write down your conclusions.

Now choose one of your older patients who has been involved with several service providers and repeat this exercise for that patient. Pay particular attention to communication issues. Try to be as objective in your assessments as you were in Mary's case, and that includes the care and communication provided by you.

SUMMARY

This chapter focused on communication. It described the component parts for ease of understanding so you can apply this knowledge when effectively communicating with older people. It discussed the reason for effective communication, what constitutes effective communication with older clients and how it can significantly aid patient satisfaction and prevent service failure. Ageing and disease can cause a loss in sensory function, such as visual loss, hearing loss and speech impairments, which seriously challenges effective communication between patient and health professional. It elaborated on these aspects, providing some useful dos and don'ts and describing some technological aids for improving communication.

Evidence clearly demonstrates that working in partnerships in a cooperative and collaborative manner is essential to quality care. Professional groups must pay attention to communication, both within their own group and with other professional groups. This chapter included the concept of working together and explained how communication can aid this process. Although often seen as a bureaucratic activity, record-keeping is an essential aspect of communication; it is the written form that should clearly articulate the assessment of the patient, the treatment regime, responses and evaluation. It is also a framework through which professionals can be more efficient and effective and it is the legal structure in which health providers can account for their actions.

◀ **Key points**

1 Effective communication in general and effective communication with older clients in particular can significantly aid patient satisfaction and prevent service failure.
2 Ageing and disease can cause a loss in sensory function, such as visual loss, hearing loss and speech impairments, which seriously challenges effective communication between patient and health professional.
3 Technology is one way to improve communication.
4 Working in partnerships in a cooperative and collaborative manner is essential to quality care.

5 Although often seen as a bureaucratic activity, record-keeping is an essential aspect of communication.

REFERENCES

Action for Dysphasic Adults (1997) *Dysphasia Matters: A Medical Teaching Pack.* Action for Dysphasic Adults, London.

Bauby, J. D. (1997) *The Diving-Bell and the Butterfly.* Fourth Estate, London.

Covey, S. (1995) *Principle-Centered Leadership.* Simon and Schuster, London.

Department of Health (1998) *Clear standards of NHS care to be set for older people for the first time.* Department of Health press release, November 1998.

D'Sa, S. (1995) Multidisciplinary bedside notes: an experiment in care. *Nursing Times*, **91**(12), 46–47.

Flaxman, K. (1997) All wrapped up? Winter admissions. *Health Service Journal*, **107**(5576), 26–27.

Forster, M. (1989) *Have the Men Had Enough?* Penguin, London.

Garwel, M. J. (1981) The effects of various drugs on speech. *British Journal of Disorders of Communication*, **16**, 1.

Gravell, R. (1988) *Communication Problems in Elderly People: Practical Approaches to Management.* Croom Helm, London.

Griffiths, H. (1991) The psychiatry of old age: the effects of dementia on communication. In: *Speech and Communication Problems in Psychiatry* (ed. Gravell, R. and Frances, J.). Chapman and Hall, London.

Health Advisory Service 2000 (1998) *Not Because They Are Old: An Independent Inquiry into the Care of Older People on Acute Wards in General Hospitals.* Health Advisory Service 2000, London.

Henwood, M. (1998) *Ignored and Invisible? Carers' Experience of the NHS. Summary of a UK Research Survey Commissioned by the Carers National Association.* Carers National Association, London.

Holmes, J., Pugner, K., Phillips, R. *et al.* (1998) Managing Alzheimer's disease: the cost of care per patient. *British Journal of Health Care Management*, **4**(7), 332–337.

Jacobs-Condit, I. (ed.) (1984) *Gerontology and Communication Disorders.* American Speech-Language-Hearing Association, Rockville MD.

Kelson, M. and Ford, C. (1998) *Stroke Rehabilitation: Patient and Carer Views.* College of Health/Royal College of Physicians, London.

Kitson, T. (1997) *Dementia Reconsidered: The Person Comes First.* Open University Press, Buckingham.

Knocker, S. (1998) Going the extra distance. *Alzheimer's Disease Society Newsletter*, 8, 8.

Langlands, A. and Moores, Y. (1999) *Making a Difference: Strengthening the Nursing, Midwifery and Health Visiting Contribution to Health and Healthcare.* NHS Executive, Leeds.

Lubinski, R., Morrison, E. and Rigrodsky, S. (1985) Perception of spoken communication by elderly chronically ill patients in institutional settings. In: *Institutionalized People: Can We Do a Better Job?* (ed. Nuru, N.). American Speech-Language-Hearing Association, Rockville MD.

Macphee, G., Crowther, J. and McAlpine, C. (1998) A simple screening test for hearing impairment in elderly patients. *Age and Ageing*, **17**, 347–351.

McCormack, P. (1997) Undernutrition in the elderly population living at home in the community: a review of the literature. *Journal of Advanced Nursing*, **26**, 5.

Miskelly, F. (2001) Assistive technology in elderly care. *Age and Ageing*, **30**, 455–458.

Nazarko, L. (1995) *Nursing in Nursing Homes.* Blackwell Science, Oxford.

Nelson-Jones, R. (1992). Personal communication. In: *Experiential Training* (ed. Hobbs, A.). Tavistock, London.

Newton, E. (1980) *This Bed My Centre*. Virago, London.

NMC (2002a) *Code of Professional Conduct*. Nursing and Midwifery Council, London.

NMC (2002b) *Guidelines for Records and Record Keeping*. Nursing and Midwifery Council, London.

Office of Population Censuses and Surveys (1999) The prevalence of disability among adults. In: *Surveys of Disability in Great Britain*. The Stationery Office, London.

Perkins, R. E. and Poynton, C. E. (1990) Group counselling for relatives of hospitalized presenile dementia patients: a controlled study. *British Journal of Clinical Psychology*, **29**(3), 287–295.

Rudat, K. (1994) *Black and Ethnic Minority Groups in England: Health and Lifestyles*. Health Education Authority, London.

Schmitt, J. F. and McCroskey, R. L. (1981) Sentence comprehension in elderly listeners: the factor of rate. *Journal of Gerontology*, **36**, 4.

Skodra, E. (1992) The lived experience of a 'stranger': reflections of a counselling psychologist working with elderly immigrant women. *Changes*, **10**(3), 197–202.

Smith, M., Rousseau, N., Lecouturier, J. *et al.* (1997) Are older people satisfied with discharge information? *Nursing Times*, **93**(43), 52–53.

Sparkes, C. (1993) The impact of language loss on marriage. *College of Speech and Language Therapists Bulletin*, **494**, 9–11.

UKCC (1999) *Practitioner–Client Relationships and the Prevention of Abuse*. United Kingdom Central Council, London.

Wahrborg, P. (1991) *Assessment and Management of Emotional and Psychosocial Reactions to Brain Damage and Aphasia*. Far Communications, Kibworth.

FURTHER READING

Websites

Age Concern: www.ageconcern.org.uk
Alzheimer's Disease Society: www.alzheimers.org.uk
Royal National Institute for the Blind: www.rnib.org.uk
Royal National Institute for the Deaf: www.rnid.org.uk

7 MULTIPLE HEALTH NEEDS OF OLDER PEOPLE

OBJECTIVES

- Define issues relating to the multiple health needs of older people.
- Discuss the risk and protective factors associated with chronic ill health.
- Explain the ways in which older people confront and cope with multiple health problems in their everyday lives.
- Identify factors that affect how older people cope with multiple health problems.
- Discuss social support as a coping strategy.
- Discuss the notion of polypharmacy and its implications for older people.
- Explain the concept of medicine management.
- Discuss the responsibility of prescribing practitioners.

INTRODUCTION

Statistical evidence suggests that when people age there is an increased probability they will develop multiple health problems of a chronic nature (Department of Health, 2001; Guralnik, 1996), which link to increasing disability and premature death (Basford *et al.*, 2003, Hoffman *et al.*, 1996). Lorig (1993) contends that people over the age of 65 years carry an average burden of approximately two conditions. Furthermore, Campbell et al. (1994) report that half of the people living in the community aged 70 years and over had impairments in more than one physiological system, including cognitive, sensory, neurological, musculoskeletal and cardiorespiratory impairments. In addition, hypertension, coronary artery disease, respiratory disease, diabetes, depression and cognitive impairment all become more prevalent with advancing age (Berman and Studenski, 1998).

With increased numbers of people reaching old age and advanced old age, it is apparent that older people will live with multiple health problems of a chronic nature. It is therefore likely that older people will make increasing demands on the health-care system and be diagnosed and treated for more than one disease. The implications of comorbidity for the patient are multifaceted and may result in social isolation, pain, loss of independence and deterioration in quality of life. As the numbers of diseases increase, there is a risk of difficulty with activities of daily living and mobility (Fried and Guralnik, 1997). Such health issues tax the individual's physical, psychological, spiritual and social well-being and can be demanding on financial resources (Poon *et al.*, 2003). The overwhelming nature of multiple health problems occupies the older person's time and energy, so much so that their daily activities often revolve around their illness and treatment regimes.

Unfortunately, once a person has developed a chronic illness, reversing the disease process is highly unlikely. Therefore the effect of the diseases can only be minimized through chronic disease management and health-promoting activities (Poon *et al.*, 2003). Thus, preventing the onset of chronic illness and comorbidity is the preferred option not only for the maintenance of health and quality of life for the individual, but also for the health and well-being of their caregivers and society. When the older person develops chronic illness and associated multiple health problems, effective coping strategies should be identified and implemented as part of the overall health management plan. Furthermore, to initiate effective coping interventions for multiple health problems, it is first necessary for health professionals to understand the nature of living with chronic illness and associated multiple pathology, the related research evidence on coping with comorbidity and life changes required to 'manage or control symptoms and potentially life threatening situations' (Basford, 2003, p. 780).

Activity

- Consider Mary's experience and identify all comorbid conditions that she has listed.
- From the case study, expand on areas other than the physical domain that may complicate her health status.
- Refer to the literature that identifies correct treatment regimes associated with her illness. Are there any known contraindications from current literature on various treatment regimes?

RISK AND PROTECTIVE FACTORS ASSOCIATED WITH CHRONIC ILL HEALTH

There is a prevailing view that as we age there is almost always a corresponding decline in physical and mental functioning. In recent times this view has been challenged given that older people are indeed heterogeneous and do not age in any degree of uniformity. Recently, research evidence supports this position and acknowledges that risks for declining health and functioning capacity at older age are influenced by lifestyle, living conditions and genetic make-up (Albert *et al.*, 1995, Basford *et al.*, 2003, Seeman *et al.*, 1995). Debates are currently focused on the need to identify risk factors that are associated with functional disability given the predominance of the oldest old having some degree of functional loss. Figure 7.1 shows a physiotherapist undertaking a risk assessment of the functional loss of an older person who has had a stroke.

Furthermore, it is questioned whether the growing population of older people will have compressed morbidity (i.e. with disease and

Figure 7.1

Risk assessment of functional loss

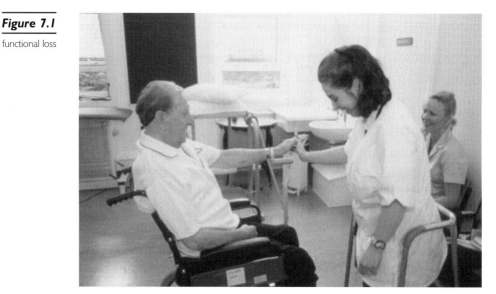

disability postponed until later ages) or whether people will live longer with multiple health problems for a greater part of their old age (Guralnik and Schneider, 1987). Seeman and Chen (2003) raise an important point as to whether the presence of major chronic illness, such as diabetes, hypertension, heart disease, cancer and fractures, is associated with declines in functioning. They state that, for the most part, scientists have focused their analysis on the older population as a whole, adjusting for various health conditions while examining the effect of lifestyle and demographic factors. By contrast, Verbrugge and Patrick (1995) have explored the impact on the levels of functioning for older people with or without chronic conditions. Their results illustrate that chronic illness has a negative association with levels of functioning.

Other studies have argued the difference that lifestyle, living conditions and personality have on health status (Penninx *et al.*, 1998b). Seeman and Chen (2003) demonstrate that older people who have chronic ill health do not necessarily suffer from loss of functioning due solely to the manifestations of the disease process; rather, their functioning is modified by lifestyle activities such as physical activity, social support, self-efficacy beliefs and psychological approaches towards life. These findings suggest that despite chronic ill health, older people can offset their loss of functional capacity by engaging in physical activities, social support and psychological stimulation. Chronic ill health is therefore not synonymous with being a burden to the individual or, indeed, society as a whole but that lifestyle and living conditions are influential factors to be considered with the older person's loss of functional capacity. Hence it is important for health professionals to address these factors when undertaking any risk assessments.

Activity

Refer back to Mary's case study and undertake a retrospective risk assessment. Map your findings with what is known about risk assessment against reduced functional capacity associated with older people.

COPING WITH MULTIPLE HEALTH CONDITIONS

In a recent systematic literature review on community-dwelling older people funded by the American Association of Retired Persons Andrus Foundation (Poon *et al.*, 2000), a list of 12 chronic health conditions was identified that had an impact on functional capacity that affected either the older person's cognitive, physical, or affective systems (Table 7.1). In each situation the effect of chronic health conditions impacts on the older person's affective and physical system with cardiovascular disease, stroke, respiratory disease and lung cancer also having an effect on cognition.

Distinguishing negative and positive coping strategies was part of the review, which was not always conclusive, given the individualistic nature of people, their culture and how they perceive their illness (Poon *et al.*, 2000). Scharloo *et al.* (1998, p. 573) comment on the structure of illness perceptions identified within the literature:

- **Identity** is the label placed on the disease and its associated symptoms.
- **Causes** are how the individual got the disease.
- **Consequences** are the expected outcomes of the disease.
- **Timescale** refers to the expectations about the perseverance and characteristics of the illness.
- **Controllability** refers to the beliefs the individual has about being able to control the disease.

Other scientists have identified coping strategies that embrace

- prevention of stress from events or situations;
- alteration of the situation or problem;
- change in the meaning of the situation;
- management of the symptoms or reaction to the stress.

In addition, Lazarus and Folkman (1984) point out that coping is a process that involves appraisal and coping concepts. Cognitive appraisal (primary appraisal) involves the individual's evaluation of the threat from internal or external stressors. If, for instance, the stressor is viewed as influencing a positive outcome, then positive emotions are more likely to result. Conversely, if the stressor is viewed negatively, this perception can damage health status on the physical and psychological self. A negative view is commonly associated with the impact of chronic health conditions. The challenge is therefore to intervene with the cycle of negativity through secondary assessment (appraisal) to determine the

Table 7.1

Prioritized list of chronic health conditions (Basford *et al*, 2000)

Rank	Disease	Cognitive	Affective	Physical	Rationale for disease	Coping rationale
1	Cardiovascular disease (CHD)	X	X	X	The estimated leading cause of mortality in the US for 1998 The estimated leading cause of death in Europe for 1998 The leading cause of work disability Some 11 million Americans aged 65 years and older report disabilities caused by CHD	Overwhelming evidence of mortality or morbidity indicates inclusion The nature of the disease (having to live with an imminent sudden attack) requires coping strategies
2	Stroke/hypertension	X	X	X	Ranked as the third most prevalent cause of death in people over 65 in the US for 1994 with 134 340 deaths Accounts for 13.7% of predicted deaths in Europe for 1998	Affects an increasing aged population in greater numbers The coping strategies required are significant, even for a mild stroke A plethora of coping strategies are raised in major stroke
3	Respiratory diseases	X (in the latter stages)	X	X	Chronic obstructive pulmonary disease (COPD) and allied conditions are the fourth most common causes of death in the US for those over 65, with 87 048 deaths	Requires coping strategies with progression of the disease process Affects cognition in later stages
4	Diabetes		X	X	Ranked as the sixth most prevalent cause of death in the US in those over 65 An estimated 16 million Americans have diabetes	If not managed, can lead to many comorbidities
5	Arthritis		X	X	Arthritis and related conditions affect nearly 43 million Americans in 1998 Nearly 50% of people over 65 have arthritis	Large prevalence of disease Leads to loss of mobility, work, hobbies At advanced stage, results in comorbidity from development of other diseases
6	Lung cancer	X (in the latter stages)	X	X	Second leading cause of work disability 14 200 predicted deaths for the over-60s Lung cancer is the leading cause of cancer-related death among men in the US	Presented symptoms are the same as for respiratory diseases but treatment is different, therefore so are coping strategies (associated with chemoradiotherapy) May affect cognition in tertiary stages of the disease and if secondary processes are involved

Table 7.1 continued

Rank	Disease	Cognitive	Affective	Physical	Rationale for disease	Coping rationale
7	Colorectal cancer		X	X	5300 predicted deaths for the over-60s Cancer of the colon or rectum is the second leading cause of cancer-related death in the US	Incidence increases with advancing age Treatment of the disease requires traumatic surgery, which requires coping strategies
8	Prostate cancer		X	X	3990 predicted deaths for males over 60 years Prostate cancer is the second most commonly diagnosed form of cancer after skin cancer among men in the US	About 80% of all men with clinically diagnosed prostate cancer fall into the age group of 65 and older Increases with age Surgical interventions require coping strategies Must cope with 'loss of manhood'
9	Breast cancer		X	X	3740 predicted deaths for women over 60 Breast cancer is the leading cancerous site in women	Incidence increases with age Surgical interventions or radiotherapy require coping strategies Radical mastectomy requires major adjustment in behaviour
10	Osteoporosis/fractures		X	X	Osteoporosis is responsible for more than 1.5 million fractures annually, including 300 000 hip fractures, 700 000 vertebral fractures, 250 000 wrist fractures, 300 000 fractures at other sites White women 65 years or older have twice the incidence of fractures as African-American women Some 10 million individuals have the disease, while 18 million have low bone mass, placing them at increased risk for osteoporosis	Results in significant mobility loss and presents problems of mortality
11	Visual impairment		X	X	For individuals aged 65 or older, the rate of blindness is 135 per 1000 In the US an estimated 15 million people are blind or visually impaired Some 70% of severely visually impaired persons are aged 65 or over	More disabling with increasing age Significant behavioural adjustments are required to cope
12	Hearing impairment		X	X	An estimated 60% of people over 65 are affected Hearing loss is the third leading chronic disability in the US	More disabling with increasing age Significant behavioural adjustments are required to cope

best course of coping intervention to be applied. This appraisal may be through problem-focused coping behavioural interventions that focus on the management of external stressors or emotion-focused coping or cognitive strategies that address emotional reactions to stress (Basford *et al.*, 2003). Martin (2003) offers another alternative coping strategy that relates to avoidance through distracting or diversion behaviour. Such coping behaviours are focused on denial and suppression and, if not addressed, can be very detrimental to health.

FACTORS THAT AFFECT COPING WITH MULTIPLE HEALTH PROBLEMS

Coping with multiple health problems is a complex phenomenon, chiefly because of the individual nature of older people. A person's individuality is nurtured and influenced by their culture and their personalities. In addition, there is an association with the older person's previous life experiences and the ways in which they cope with illness. For example, if a person had never had a debilitating illness, their coping experience would be limited. However, if older people have experienced ill health as a child and young adult, then they will have adopted coping strategies (negative or positive) to help them through their illness. These coping strategies become internalized and drawn upon in subsequent illnesses, consciously or unconsciously. Other factors that affect coping with multiple health problems relate to gender, education, compliance with therapeutic interventions or professional advice, and age differences.

Brown and Nicassio (1987) highlight the coping differences between the genders, particularly that women have a more positive reappraisal than men, whereas Folkman *et al.* (1987) suggest that men use more self-control by keeping their feelings to themselves. The level of an individual's educational attainment is a significant factor in the use of negative or positive coping strategies. de Klerk *et al.* (1997) have shown that a low level of education has a correlation with the use of inappropriate coping behaviours. Supporting this concept, Verbrugge *et al.* (1991) identified that fewer years in education often results in greater disability throughout one's life. Non-compliance with therapeutic interventions or professional advice is associated with negative coping strategies. Factors that assist in compliant behaviour are linked to social support, knowledge of the disease, partnerships working between clients and professional agents, and mastery of self-management as in the case of diabetes (MacLean and Lo, 1998). Age differences can affect how individuals cope with health problems. Those who are more advanced in years adopt a more philosophical stance, use less hostility and escapism, and often adopt the use of management strategies rather than coping strategies, i.e. older people become adept at circumnavigating their problems through the use of effective management strategies (Aldwin *et al.*, 1996).

Coping strategies used with chronic health conditions fall into three domains – cognitive, physical and affective – or a combination of all three. Some of these strategies will support a negative health outcome and others a positive health outcome. Those of a negative disposition relate to confrontational behaviour, defensiveness, pessimism, certain types of social support, fatalism, emotive behaviour, taking abusive substances, self-blame, withdrawal and catastrophizing. Positive coping strategies are focused on the patient having high-self esteem, mastery of the situation, the ability to self-manage, and a strong belief in cure and religiosity (Basford *et al.*, 2003).

SOCIAL FACTORS AFFECTING COPING

The significance of social support should not be underestimated as a coping strategy used by older people, given that people live and work within a social framework. Within this framework, health of individuals is supported through reciprocal arrangements, usually within the family, or kinship arrangements. When individuals succumb to illness, care and support are often given as a sense of duty within societal expectations and social policy (Department of Health, 1990). From this premise, there is an assumption that social support is given willingly, but the reality is very different for older people who need long-term sustained care. In this instance the experience is not always positive, because many caregivers feel resentment towards their loved ones (Sarason *et al.*, 1990). Nonetheless, scientists have established that there is an intricate relationship between health and social support and this relationship has had a positive correlation in reducing morbidity and premature mortality (Berkman *et al.*, 1992; Felton, 1990; Nissen and Newman, 1992).

Furthermore, social support enables people to cope better with chronic illness and emotional stress (Felton, 1990; Penninx *et al.*, 1998a). However, social support is a complex phenomenon in that it defies a uniform definition. Accordingly, Hutchinson (1999) proclaims that it is a 'meta concept' which precludes a consensus of opinion being reached. There is also a difference between social support and social networks. Social support may be defined in terms of social networks that embrace the notion of accessibility of support to an individual through social ties, groups and the community. The two concepts are seen as separate, whereas in another sense, they are viewed as an inter-related whole. Cohen and Willis (1985) attempted to clarify this position by suggesting that social support is concerned with quality indicators or functional contexts of relationships, and social networks relate specifically to the number and various dimensions associated with these relationships. Cohen and Syme (1985) point out that attention should be given to the type of support and its relationship to need, at the point of need, and throughout the whole duration of need. They continue to suggest that perceptions of support given should be explored to illustrate if perceived need reflects met need. Indeed, the unravelling of social support is a complex issue and some researchers have suggested it should be examined within a taxonomy framework that may best identify and differentiate between the following categories: social integration, network resource, supportive climate and environment, received and enacted support, and perception of being supported.

While the debate continues over the nuances and definitions of social support, it is widely accepted that, in the context of the illness paradigm, social support as a coping strategy has a positive health outcome and can effectively enhance quality of life and reduce morbidity and premature mortality. The main thread to the argument is that social support is instrumental in influencing behavioural changes that lead to a 'healthy lifestyle' and can be most effective when associated with illness. To illustrate this concept, Ruberman *et al.* (1984) explored the effects of social isolation and its impact on recovery after a myocardial infarction. Among the 2320 male survivors who participated in the study, the main issues arising were that (i) cognitive ability was stimulated through the educational process and (ii) having social support did have a positive correlation with staving off premature mortality.

Such a position is supported by Welin *et al.* (1992), who point out that there is a reduced mortality with individuals who have cancer, coronary heart disease and coronary vascular disease. The reason for this phenomenon is not yet clearly understood but there are suggestions that it is because of behavioural changes such as smoking cessation, reduction in alcohol consumption, healthier dietary intake, the utilization of health services, health education and social and economic aid (Penninx *et al.*, 1998a). The mediating effect of social support with premature death is of significance but consideration should also be given to the notion that the lack of social support also has a direct relationship with psychological distress and illness (Kaplan *et al.*, 1977). Confronted with the effects of a chronic illness and multiple health problems, the older person can become increasingly isolated from society, thereby seriously jeopardizing their quality of life. It is therefore incumbent on health professionals to seek ways in which positive social support can be engineered for (i) older people who have limited social networks and support systems or (ii) in social relationships that impact negatively on their health.

MEDICINES AND OLDER PEOPLE

Older people more often take multiple drugs for their multiple diseases. In 1998 the Health Survey for England identified that 36% of people aged 75 years were taking four or more prescribed drugs. Polypharmacy (i.e. taking four or more prescribed drugs) is a major risk factor for older people due to the potential for adverse drug reactions, increased risk of drug interaction, readmission to hospital due to non-compliance or adverse drug reaction, and increased risk of falls. One of the effects of the ageing process, particularly if there are multiple health problems, is that the clearance of drugs through elimination is reduced. Therefore, for most medicines, the margin between therapeutic dose and toxic dose becomes narrower than for people with full functional capacity. If the older person's health situation is further exacerbated by acute illness, the situation may lead to high concentrations of medications in the tissues. Of particular note are hypnotics, diuretics and non-steroidal anti-inflammatory drugs (NSAIDs). According to the British National Formulary, these drugs are often associated with significantly reducing the blood pressure (hypotension), increasing the likelihood of falls (hypnotics and diuretics), and internal bleeding (NSAIDs) in older people.

Without a doubt, prescribing medications is the most frequent clinical intervention that follows the traditional medical model. The finances associated with this practice relate to more than 50% of the total NHS budget. In addition, older people receive 50% of all prescription items, of which 78% are repeat prescriptions (Royal College of Physicians, 1997). With the advancement of age, there is an increased likelihood that multiple health problems will prevail and increase an older person's dependency on medications to sustain life and, hopefully, improve the quality of life. For example, in nursing homes or residential care homes, older people are at higher risk of medication-related problems given that they will receive up to four times as many prescription items compared to older people who live in their own home (Walley and Scott, 1995) and, furthermore, they are prescribed six to seven drugs per person (Furniss *et al.*, 1998). Furniss *et al.* (1998) also point out that older people in nursing homes required modifications to treatment with the most frequent recommended action (47%) to stop all medications. Furthermore, in two-thirds of these cases, there was no clinical evidence for the prescribed medication. On follow-up it was identified that modification of treatments had no adverse effect on morbidity and mortality (Furniss *et al.*, 1998).

Although this section has focused on prescribed medication, for many older adults their chronic illnesses are all too often incurable. Thus, because prescribed medicines do not always effectively manage their symptoms, older people often turn to over-the-counter drugs bought from local stores, pharmacies or herbalists. Such combinations of 'drug cocktails' can stimulate adverse reactions to the detriment of people's health and well-being. It is therefore important that older people should be the greatest beneficiaries of appropriate and optimal drug treatment, which encourages a positive health outcome and negates the need to purchase over-the-counter drugs. For the most part, assessing an individual's total medication intake (prescribed and non-prescribed) is all too often overlooked and, if unchecked, can be extremely damaging to the health of the older person. Therefore, when undertaking a health assessment, it is essential that these extraneous medications or treatments are considered and documented as part of the assessment process.

Over the past few decades there has been increasing concern given to the appropriateness of prescribing medicines to older people arising from the increased susceptibility older people have to iatrogenic diseases caused by inappropriate treatment regimes, incorrect medication and inadequate monitoring of drug therapy. In addition, the complexity of the treatment regime often supports non-compliance because of the person's inability to self-manage the process. The *National Service Framework for Older People* (Department of Health, 2001) has embraced this notion and has proclaimed that all older people have the right to 'the right medicine, at the right dose and in the right form' (p. 1). This was written in recognizing that older people do have serious negative health outcomes through the improper prescribing of medicines. Several studies show that an adverse reaction to drugs is a common cause of hospital admission (Cunningham *et al.*, 1997; Mannesse *et al.*, 2000) and, while in hospital, 6–17% of older in-patients experience adverse drug reactions (Mannesse *et al.*, 2000). In addition, Mannesse *et al.* (2000) highlight the fact that older people are not always prescribed drugs that would be of benefit against stroke or asthma, antidepressants, and antithrombotic treatments.

It is also suggested that older people may not be as compliant with the taking of prescribed drugs due to complex regimes, diminished cognitive ability or lack of knowledge and understanding. The Royal College of Physicians (2000) demonstrated that up to 25% of medicines were prescribed 'as required' or 'take as directed', which lacks any degree of specificity. To address the anomalies and poor prescribing practices, policy makers advocate a new model for managing medicines within the NHS. The main focus of the model is partnership working to include colleagues, older people as patients and their caregivers.

Medicines management

Managing medicines within complex organizations such as the NHS brings certain challenges. For example, there are two distinct philosophies between primary and secondary care. Primary care reflects

> *the systematic provision of medicines therapy through a partnership of effort between patients and professionals to deliver best patient outcomes at minimized cost. (Tweedie and Jones, 2001)*

Secondary care suggests that

> *medicines management in hospitals encompasses the entire way that medicines are selected, procured, delivered, prescribed, administered and reviewed to optimize the contribution that medicines make to producing informed and desired outcomes of patient care. (Audit Commission, 2001)*

Despite the philosophical differences, there are some common elements, chiefly (i) helping people to get the most from their medicines to maintain or increase their quality and duration of life, (ii) ensuring people do not suffer from iatrogenic illness due to inappropriate therapy, (iii) medication prescription is optimized early in the treatment regime, (iv) supporting and empowering patients in the use of their medicines, and (v) reducing drug waste.

Partnership working is a key theme of the NHS Plan, which is designed to empower people to take an active role in managing their own health care. Patients and clients are no longer passive recipients in medicines prescribing, but take on an active role in prescribing decisions. Their beliefs and cultural norms are considered given that these factors influence people's knowledge and understanding with regard to 'how medicines work and how they are best used' (Department of Health, 2001, p. 20). Moreover, in meeting the need for compliance, drug regimes must meet the normal schedules of daily life. Current working models fall short of this ideal, with little or no dialogue existing between health-care professionals in primary and secondary care facilities. Indeed there is evidence that changes to medication protocols on discharge are made by the GP without always having the clinical evidence to back up the decision (Department of Health, 1998). These decisions often include restarting medicines that were stopped in hospital and duplication of medication treatment using generic and branded drugs (Department of Health, 2001, p. 8).

Moreover, there is a lack of coordinated planning and effective communication between primary and hospital care that would reduce the delay of medications and significantly improve the continuity of care within and between organizations (Duffin *et al.*, 1998). Duggan *et al.* (1998) suggest that pharmaceutical discrepancies can be halved if the discharge prescription regime is sent to the community pharmacy as well as the GP. Repeat medications are all too often unnecessary, ineffective and inappropriate; have no routine monitoring; and often encourage non-compliance. Clearly it is the responsibility of all health professionals to monitor the effects of medication and assess the potential role that drugs may have had in causing symptoms in the first place. Table 7.2 sets out barriers to medicines management reviews and some opportunities. The Department of Health (2001) suggests that with 'any adverse change in health such as confusion and dizziness [the patient's] medicines should be reviewed' (p. 9). The document identifies the medication review format:

- Explanation of the purpose of the review and the reason why periodic review is important.
- Compilation of the list of medicines taken or used with the list of medicines prescribed.
- Comparison of the list of medicines taken or used with the list of medicines prescribed.
- The patient's (and caregiver's) own perception and understanding of the purpose of the medication, and any misconceptions.
- The patient's (and caregiver's) understanding of how much, how often and when medicines should be taken.
- Application of prescribing appropriateness indicators (e.g. the

Table 7.2

Medicine management reviews

Barriers or challenges	Opportunities
Professional dominance	Synergistic approaches towards information management technology
Time constraints	Hand-held and electronic patient records
Historical practices of communication	Integrated working models between health and social care
Lack of patient-held records	One-stop dispensing
Lack of clear and concise admission and discharge information	Dissemination of best practice
Increasing number of independent prescribers	Working and learning together
Lack of electronic compatibility and/or electronic resources	

indication for the drug is recorded and upheld by the British National Formulary).

- Have any side effects been experienced? Evidence suggests that older people's accounts of perceived side effects correlate closely with health professionals' assessments. The review should include social side effects, which restrict people's lifestyles (e.g. wakefulness at night or excessive diuresis affecting social life). Are some medicines being used to treat side effects of other medications?
- Review of any relevant monitoring tests (e.g. INR for patients on anticoagulants, Hb1Ac for diabetic patients, blood tests for disease-modifying antirheumatic drugs, thyroid hormone levels).

Activity

- Read the document *Pharmacy in the Future – Implementing the NHS Plan: A Programme for Pharmacy in the National Health Service* (Department of Health, 2000).
- Identify the reasons why partnerships in pharmacy are necessary.
- At what operational level will this model be applied?
- Identify any published documents that refer to partnership in pharmacy or related concepts.
- Reflect on your organization's medicine policy and model for practice.
- Reflect on Mary's case study and identify any issues around pharmacy.

FUTURE CHALLENGES IN MEDICINES MANAGEMENT

Developing partnerships with other professional colleagues and the patient and their carer requires a phenomenal culture shift for all parties concerned. Having experienced a patriarchal approach towards health-care provision throughout the life of the NHS, it is not easy to develop partnerships, it is not easy to help empower an older person and it is not easy for the older person to accept joint ownership. Besides these difficulties, there are other challenges to consider:

- The need for more meaningful communication, coordination and collaboration between primary and secondary care providers. For example, records of prescribing and information relating to compliance or administration issues on admission plus clear and relevant medication information on discharge, which is shared by all parties, including the patient and carer. Ideally there should be a single electronic record.
- NHS trust clinical governance development plans need to address quality assurance and monitoring procedures related to medicines management.
- Shared care guidelines need to be further developed to ensure there is a transparent approach to local prescribing decisions.
- The development of a patient-held record, which identifies current medicines regimes, allergies and administration problems and allows pharmacists, nurses and others to provide adequate support for the patient. This process should form part of the single assessment framework.
- To provide a patient-centred service, there is a need to increase the number of prescribers and improve the methods of obtaining medications, making both more accessible to older people. This suggestion involves the extension of nurses prescribing and improving access through walk-in centres or NHS Direct. In addition, this plan should involve the introduction of pharmacy prescribing and new ways of working to deliver pharmacy services to support patients and their carers in managing medicines.
- Essential improvements to repeat-prescribing systems include protocols for issuing and reviewing patients' medication regimes, systems that target patients at higher risk of medication problems, and recording or linking of all medicines issued to patients at different times and locations.
- Improved access is necessary to the pharmacy or the surgery and there should be a medicine collection and delivery service.

Although these intentions are laudable, health practitioners must be mindful that the NHS still needs to decide on priorities to meet the

By 2002	All people over 75 years should normally have their medicines reviewed annually and those taking four or more medicines should be reviewed every six months (Department of Health, 2001)
By 2002	All hospitals should have a 'one-stop dispensing/dispensing for discharge' scheme and, where appropriate, self-administration schemes for medicines for older people (Department of Health, 2001)
By 2002	A leadership programme will deliver 30 leaders in each of medicine, nursing, and pharmacy (Joint Task Force on Patient Partnership in Medicine Taking)
By 2004	Every PCT across the country will have schemes so that people get more help from pharmacists in using their medicines (Department of Health, 2000)
By 2004	Expert patient pilot schemes will cover all PCT sites (Department of Health, 2001)
By 2007	Expert patient programmes will be mainstreamed throughout the NHS (Department of Health, 2001)

Table 7.3

Primary care trusts: some key milestones

conflicting demands of older people. However, this requirement should not stop progress in medicines management and should have the added value of being effective, efficient and economical. In pursuit of these aims, Table 7.3 (page 183) identifies some key delivery milestones for the primary care trusts (PCTs).

The responsibility of prescribing practitioners

Until recently medical doctors and dentists were the only two professional groups who could legally prescribe medicines. Two factors drive the challenge to this monopoly: the need to maximize benefit to patients and the preference of the NHS to increase flexible use of workforce skills. What has subsequently evolved is a broader way for health professionals to prescribe within their scope or field of practice (Table 7.4). The mechanisms for prescribing are through patient group directives, nurse prescribing (extended formulary) and supplementary prescribing (nurses and pharmacists).

Table 7.4	Patient group directives	Health Service Circular (HSC2000/026) August 2000 (Colin Pearson)
History and legislation: supply and prescribing	Extended formulary: nurse prescribing	POM Order Amendment, April 2002
		NHS Pharmaceutical Regulatory Changes, April 2002
	Supplementary prescribing	Health and Social Care Act, May 2001; Regulations, April 2003

Who can use a patient group directive?

The registered health professionals who can prescribe under a patient group directive are nurses, midwives, health visitors, ambulance paramedics, optometrists, chiropodists, radiographers, orthoptists, physiotherapists and pharmacists. The definition of a patient group directive is 'a written instruction for the supply or administration of medicines to groups of patients who may not be individually identified before presentation of treatment' (Department of Health, 2003). The majority of clinical care should be on an individual, patient-specific basis and the directive must be signed by a senior doctor (or dentist) and a senior pharmacist.

Independent prescribing by nurses

Apart from doctors and dentists, nurses were the first professional group to be independent prescribers. However, this prescribing role was limited initially to district nurses and health visitors who had undergone further education and training. The formulary from which they could independently prescribe was limited and related to appliances, dressings and a few medicines. This model of practice was evaluated and found to benefit the patients, even though it was limited in practice. What then transpired was the development of the extended formulary for nurse prescribers, which allowed suitably educated nurses to prescribe for minor illnesses, minor surgery, health promotion, and palliative care within their field of practice.

Following in the footsteps of extended nurse prescribing was the notion of supplementary prescribing that enables nurses and pharmacists to prescribe. This is perceived to assist in continuing care and chronic disease management such as diabetes, asthma and hypertension. Supplementary prescribing is defined as 'a voluntary prescribing partnership between the Independent Prescriber and a Supplementary Prescriber, to implement an agreed patient-specific Clinical Management Plan with the patient's agreement' (Department of Health, 2003). It is hypothesized that, with the right safeguards in place, supplementary prescribing will increase efficiency and effectiveness of care and will have the added value of increasing teamworking and skill mix. For such a plan to work, it is suggested there should be a written clinical management plan specific to a named patient and the patient's health condition. There are no legal restrictions on supplementary prescribing except for controlled drugs (for now) and unlicensed medicines, unless within clinical trials or with an exemption certificate. Table 7.5 lists the principles to support supplementary prescribing.

Patient safety is of paramount importance
There must be benefit to the patient and the NHS
Team management of medicines must be through patient agreement
There must be effective communication between all prescribers and reciprocal access to the patient's record
There must be voluntary partnership and the separation of prescribing and dispensing responsibilities where possible

Table 7.5

Principles to support supplementary prescribing

Extending prescribing practice to other professional groups has extended the scope of professional practice and professional responsibility and accountability. Such role expansion is set to continue into the foreseeable future. This requires attention to education and training to ensure health-care practitioners are competent and fit to practise.

SUMMARY

The complexity that underpins the care of older people who have multi-dimensional health problems has meant a rethink in the ways that the health and social care services are organized and delivered. Part of health and social care reforms is to redress the weaknesses in the current organizational frameworks that have evolved since the beginnings of the NHS. It is evident from repeated service failure with older people that the system fails to offer a quality service to all. Indeed the medical model has focused on services that have centred on single-disease entities (diabetes, coronary heart disease, stroke, etc.), without due consideration that the health needs of many older people are multi-faceted and require a different knowledge base and approach to care interventions. Retaining historical working practices did not always benefit patients and their caregivers, so new models of partnership working have been encouraged through policy and legislation. This decision has allowed professional groups such as nurses to take the lead role in managing care, particularly in the fields of chronic disease management, continuing care and health promotion. Along with these changes is the need for nurses and others to ensure that they practise from an evidence base and that they understand their professional accountability to older people and also their professional colleagues.

Key points ▶

1 From reading the evidence it is clear that the health needs of older people are somewhat different from those of other age groups.

2 Older people are more susceptible to multiple health problems and are challenged to effectively apply coping strategies that at least maintain their health status throughout the duration of chronic illness.

3 It is a professional responsibility to assess for risks and apply protective factors wherever possible. Within this context it is also the duty of health professionals to work in partnerships not only through the period of assessment and diagnosis but also within the frameworks of medicines management and prescribing practice.

4 The development of extending prescribing practice beyond doctors and dentists has influenced role expansion and role changes, especially when caring for older people.

REFERENCES

Albert, M. S., Jones, K., Savage, C. R., Berkman, L., Seeman, T. and Blazer, D. (1995) Predictions of cognitive change in older persons: the McArthur studies of successful aging. *Psychology and Aging*, **10**, 578–589.

Aldwin, C. M., Sutton, K. J., Chiara, G. and Spiro, A. (1996) Age difference in stress, coping and appraisal: findings from normative aging study. *Journal of Gerontology*, **51B**, 179–188.

Audit Commission (2001) *A Spoonful of Sugar – Medicine Management in NHS Hospitals*. Audit Commission, London.

Basford, L. (2003) Gerontological nursing. In: *Theory and Practice of Nursing: An Integrated Approach to Caring Practice 2nd edition* (ed. Basford, L. and Slevin, O.). Nelson Thornes, Cheltenham, Glos., pp. 775–790.

Basford C., Dowzer, C., Booth, A. and Poon, L. W. (2000) *Living with Multiple Chronic Health Conditions: A Systematic Search and Literature Review*. Final Report for the American Association of Retired Persons.

Basford, L., Poon, L. W., Dowzer, C. and Booth, A. (2003) Coping with specific chronic health conditions. In: *Successful Aging and Adaptation with Chronic Diseases* (ed. Poon, L., Hall-Gueldner, S. and Sprouse, B. M.). Springer, New York.

Berkman, L. F., Leo-Summers, L. and Horwitz, R. I. (1992) Emotional support and survival after myocardial infarction: a prospective, population-based study of the elderly. *Annals of Internal Medicine*, **177**(12), 1003–1009.

Berman, A. and Studenski, S. (1998) Musculoskeletal rehabilitation. *Clinics in Geriatric Medicine*, **14**(3), 641–659.

Brown, G. K. and Nicassio, P. M. (1987) Development of a questionnaire for the assessment of active and passive coping strategies in chronic pain patients. *Pain*, **31**, 53–64.

Campbell, A. J., Bushy, W. J., Robertson, M. C., Lum, C. L., Langlois, J. A. and Morgan, F. C. (1994) Disease, impairment, disability and social handicap: a community based study of people aged 70 years and over. *Disability and Rehabilitation* **16**(2), 72–79.

Cohen, S. and Syme, S. (1985) Issues in the study and application of social support. In: *Social Support and Health*. Academic Press, Orlando FL.

Cohen, S. and Willis, T. (1985) Stress and social support and the buffering hypothesis. *Psychological Bulletin*, **98**(2), 310–357.

Cunningham, G., Dodd, T. R. P., Grant, D. J., McMurdo, M. and Richards, R. M. E. (1997) Drug-related problems in elderly patients admitted to Tayside hospitals, methods for prevention and subsequent reassessment. *Age and Ageing*, **26**, 375–382.

de Klerk, M. M. Y, Huijsmann, R. and McDonnell, J. (1997) The use of technical aids for elderly persons in the Netherlands: an application of the Anderson and Newman model. *Gerontologist*, **37**(3), 365–373.

Department of Health (1990) *Community Care Act*. The Stationery Office, London.

Department of Health (1998) *Health Survey for England*. The Stationery Office, London.

Department of Health (2000) *Pharmacy in the Future – Implementing the NHS Plan: A Programme for Pharmacy in the National Health Service*. The Stationery Office, London.

Department of Health (2001) *National Service Framework for Older People*. The Stationery Office, London.

Department of Health (2003) *Extending Prescribing Responsibilities – Supplementary Prescribing*. The Stationery Office, London.

Duffin, J., Norwood, J. and Blenkinsopp, A. (1998) An investigation into medication changes initiated in general practice after patients are discharged from hospital. *Pharmacology Journal*, supplement to Volume 261.

Duggan, C., Feldman, R., Hough, J. and Bates, I. (1998) Reducing adverse prescribing discrepancies following hospital discharge. *International Journal of Pharmacy Practice*, **6**, 77–82.

Felton, B. J. (1990) Coping and social support in older people's experiences of chronic illness. In: *Stress and Coping in Later Life* (ed. Stephens, M., Parris A. and Crowther, J. H. E.). Hemisphere, New York, pp. 153–171.

Folkman, S., Lazarus, R. S., Pimley, S. and Novacek, J. (1987) Age differences in stress and coping processes. *Psychology of Aging*, **2**(2), 171–184.

Fried, L. P. and Guralnik, J. M. (1997) Disability in older adults: evidence regarding significance, etiology, and risk. *Journal of the American Geriatrics Society*, **45**(1), 92–100.

Furniss, L., Craig, S. K. L. and Burns, A. (1998) Medication use in nursing homes for elderly people. *International Journal of Geriatric Psychiatry*, **13**, 433–439.

Guralnik, J. M. (1996) Assessing the impact of comorbidity in the older population. *Annals of Epidemiology*, **6**, 376–380.

Guralnik, J. M. and Schneider, E. L. (1987) The compression of morbidity: a dream which may come true, someday. *Gerontologica Perspecta*, **1**, 8–14.

Hoffman, C., Rice, P. and Sung, H. Y. (1996) Persons with chronic conditions: their prevalence and costs. *Journal of the American Medical Association*, **276**(18), 1473–1479.

Hutchinson, C. (1999) Social support: factors to consider when designing studies that measure social support. *Journal of Advanced Nursing*, **29**(6), 1520–1526.

Kaplan, B. H., Cassel, J. C. and Gore, S. (1977) Social support and health. *Medical Care*, **15**, 47–50.

Lazarus, R. S. and Folkman, S. (1984) *Stress, Appraisal and Coping*. Springer, New York.

Lorig, K. (1993) Self-management of chronic illness: a model for the future. *Generations*, **17**(3), 11–14.

MacLean, D. and Lo, R. (1998) The non-insulin-dependent diabetic: success and failure in compliance. *Australian Journal of Advanced Nursing*, **14**(4), 33–42.

Mannesse, C. K., Derkx, R. H., de Ridder, M. A., Man in't Veld, A. J. and van der Cammen, T. J. (2000) Contribution of adverse drug reactions to hospital admission of older patients. *Age and Ageing*, **29**, 35–39.

Martin, P. (2003) Coping with multiple chronic health conditions. In: *Successful Aging and Adaptation with Chronic Diseases* (ed. Poon, L., Hall-Gueldner, S. and Sprouse, B. M.). Springer, New York.

Nissen, S. J. and Newman, W. P. (1992) Factors influencing reintegration to normal living after amputation. *Archives of Physical Medicine and Rehabilitation*, **73**(6), 548–551.

Penninx, B. W. J. H., vanTilburg, J., Boeke, A. J. P., Deeg, D. J. H., Kriegsman, D. M. W. and vanEijk, J. T. M. (1998a) Effects of social support and personal coping resources on depressive symptoms: different for various chronic health conditions. *Health Psychology*, **17**, 551–558.

Penninx, B. W. J. H., vanTilburg, J., Kriegsman, D. M. W., Deeg, D. J. H., Boeke, A. J. P. and Van Eijk, J. T. M. (1998b) Effects of social support and personal coping resources on mortality in older age: the longitudinal aging study in Amsterdam. *American Journal of Epidemiology*, **146**, 510–519.

Poon, L. W., Basford, L., Hall-Gueldner, S., Douzer, C., Booth, A., Penrod, J., Loeb, S. and Falkerstem, S. (2000) *Living with Multiple Chronic Health Conditions: Andrus Foundation Final Report*. University of Georgia Gerontological Centre, Athens GA.

Poon, L. W., Basford, L., Douzer, C. and Booth, A. (2003) Coping with comorbidity. In: *Successful Aging and Adaptation with Chronic Diseases* (ed. Poon, L., Hall-Gueldner, S. and Sprouse, B. M.). Springer, New York.

Royal College of Physicians (1997) *Medication for Older People*, 2nd edn. Royal College of Physicians, London.

Royal College of Physicians (2000) *National Sentinel Clinical Audit of Evidence-Based Prescribing for Older People*. Royal College of Physicians, London.

Ruberman, W., Weinblatt, E., Goldberg, J. D. and Chaudhary, B. S. (1984) Psychosocial influences on mortality after myocardial infarction. *New England Journal of Medicine*, **311**(9), 552–559.

Sarason, B. R., Sarason, I. G. and Pierce, G. R. (1990) Traditional views of social support and their impact on assessment. In: *Social Support: An International View* (ed. Sarason, B. R., Sarason, I. G. and Pierce, G. R.). Wiley, New York, pp. 7–25.

Scharloo, M., Kaptein, A. A., Weinman, J., Hazes, J. M., Willems, L., Bergman, W. and Rooijmans, H. G. (1998) Illness perceptions, coping and functioning in patients with rheumatoid arthritis, chronic obstructive pulmonary disease and psoriasis. *Journal of Psychosomatic Research*, **44**(5), 573–585.

Seeman, T. and Chen, X. (2003) Risk and protective factors for physical functioning in older adults with or without chronic conditions: the McArthur studies of successful aging. In: *Successful Aging and Adaptation with Chronic Diseases* (ed. Poon, L., Hall-Gueldner, S. and Sprouse, B. M.). Springer, New York.

Seeman, T. E., Berkman, L. F., Charpentier, P., Blazer, D., Albert, M. and Tinetti, M. (1995) Behavioural and psychosocial predictors of physical performance: the McArthur studies of successful aging. *Journal of Gerontology*, **50A**, M177–M183.

Tweedie, L. and Jones, K. (2001) *Developing patient care: medicine management in community pharmacy*. Pharmaceutical Services Negotiating Committee.

Verbrugge, L. M., Gates, D. M. and Ike, R. N. (1991) Risk factors for disability among US adults with arthritis. *Journal of Clinical Epidemiology*, **44**, 167–182.

Verbrugge, L. M. and Patrick, D. L. (1995) Seven chronic conditions: their impact on US adults activity levels and use of medical service. *American Journal of Public Health*, **85**, 173–182.

Walley, T. and Scott, A. K. (1995) Prescribing in the elderly. *Postgrad Medical Journal*, **71**, 466–471.

Welin, L., Larsson, B., Svardsudd, K., Tibbins, B. and Tibbins, G. (1992) Social network and activities in relation to mortality from cardiovascular disease, cancer and other causes: a 12 year follow-up of the study of men born in 1913 and 1923. *Journal of Epidemiology Community Health*, **46**, 127–132.

8 FORWARD TO THE FUTURE: LEADING AND MANAGING CHANGE

OBJECTIVES

- Describe the future influences in health care from institutional, national and international perspectives.
- Describe specific trends that directly affect the health and social care of older people.
- Identify and briefly describe three types of change.
- Describe two models of change.
- Identify and briefly describe six factors influencing change within health-care settings.
- Describe four requirements of leadership for successful management of health-care arenas.
- Explain the role of health-care professionals in managing change.
- Discuss three research initiatives of the Department of Health that support the future of health care.

INTRODUCTION

In considering health care for older people, we must be informed by the past and we must re-evaluate the present so that we can go forward into the future with a degree of knowledge and understanding. Without having a crystal ball, this is the most logical approach as it pre-empts the need for reactive responses to situations and allows for a smooth, planned transition into the future.

In the previous century we witnessed and celebrated the dawn of an ageing society. It is arguably a point in human history of monumental importance to all society, given the huge potential to stabilize global power and global economy. The premise is that the wisdom inherent in the collective aged population would address inequalities with compassion, knowledge and understanding of the needs and rights of all people. Conversely, the doomsayers contend that an ageing population will continue to be a burden on society; it will create an imbalance of world power and continue the unequal distribution of the global economy. Inevitably, the jury is still out on what will manifest, but if we believe the doomsayers, we should be mindful that in western societies not only do we have an increased ageing population, we also have the lowest birth rate. This situation currently concerns politicians, epidemiologists and others responsible for determining population trends plus their impact on the economy, health and social care.

However, we have a situation where the highest birth rates are enjoyed by countries that have weak economies. If these trends continue, the picture will change dramatically in the next few decades, in that there will be a greater need for multicultural harmony, global markets that sustain human needs, and a more balanced distribution of wealth and natural resources. Furthermore, the situation will be influenced by the increased mobility of populations, due to increased travel opportunities, climate changes, work, war, famine and natural disasters. It is therefore hypothesized that there will be a significant shift in multi-genealogy within and between nations. Currently nations are inextricably entwined with each other, politically and economically, supporting the notion that we are a global village interconnected and interrelated on many dimensions that include manufacturing, food chains and the provision of health care. These trends cannot easily be reversed and will continue into the immediate future.

Given these frameworks, it is with good reason that politicians, epidemiologists, health and social care professionals and others have given due attention to the effects of an ageing society. Historians have explained the phenomenon of ageing populations from the improvements in social welfare, the environment in which we live and work, scientific discoveries, therapeutic advancements, technology, health promotion and a raising of a collective consciousness towards older people. The impact that these developments and initiatives have had on the health and social care professions is indeed remarkable, and if these trends continue, which is expected, then the future will be even more challenging and demanding.

As a result of these trends, the health-care system today is fraught with change. Indeed it is often noted that change is the only constant factor within health-care arenas. This focus on change is understandable given the advances in scientific discovery, medicine and technology that directly affect the diagnostic potential, treatment regimes and delivery of health care. Concomitantly, leaders within health-care institutions view this constant change as an opportunity to continually improve health-care services. Working within a constantly changing environment requires individuals who can provide exemplary leadership.

Leadership is integral to resolving complex problems that tend to arise within health and social care environments. Effective leaders employ their knowledge, skills and attitudes to create an organizational climate in which all employees share common values, beliefs and commitment to providing quality health-care services. Leaders achieve their goals by ensuring a vision of the possible, gaining and supporting a strong team of health-care professionals to attain goals and fostering the development of all members of the health-care team while remaining receptive to expected and unexpected factors that require a change in plans or goals.

Health-care professionals also recognize that factors affecting their practice originate at various levels, such as local, national and international. Some of these factors demand a change in policy and ultimately practice. Furthermore, health-care professionals acknowledge that solutions require creative and critical thinking as well as currency in knowledge and competences to keep abreast of institutional, governmental and global issues and the ensuing change.

SIGNIFICANT ROLES IN CHANGE

Change refers to an ongoing process whereby there is an intention to alter something from a current state to a new state. Change is constant in all aspects of life today and is especially challenging when individuals confront change within their work settings. Skelton-Green (1999) describes three types of change: developmental, spontaneous and planned. The first type, developmental change, occurs as an organization grows and increases in complexity. As an example, hospital administrators may create a new programme with specialized, albeit limited, service. Within a short period of time, the programme's success and community need for services demand that administrators consider expansion of the programme. This expansion of services may or may not be planned, but organization administrators respond to the increased demand for services.

Spontaneous change requires reaction to circumstances beyond the control of the organization. A typical unexpected situation might be weather related (e.g. tornado, hurricane, heat wave, snowstorm). For instance, a heavy snowstorm often results in a series of car accidents, which requires hospitalization of numerous seriously ill patients. Skelton-Green states, 'Successful responses to spontaneous change require flexibility, cohesiveness, and a level of trust within the organization' (*ibid.*, p. 459). Planned change refers to those activities that are intentionally directed to identifying shortcomings, creating solutions and implementing steps to achieve a desired alternative approach to practice. Planned change occurs at all levels of an organization. On a nursing unit, for instance, planned change might include activities associated with implementing a self-scheduling model of staffing compared to the matron developing staffing schedules monthly.

There are several models of change in the literature. Kurt Lewin's (1951) model has three phases: unfreezing, moving and refreezing. In the unfreezing phase, the problem requiring change is identified. Lewin suggests that a force-field analysis is necessary to assess driving and restraining forces. Ideally this information is shared with all stakeholders for determining the appropriate steps to resolve the problem. This group may then develop a plan to achieve the desired results, that is, to correct the problem. There is an inherent need to reduce the factors restricting the planned change and to enhance the factors supporting the planned change. The actions to realize the new practice are implemented during the moving phase. The refreezing phase reflects the stabilizing of the new practice to the extent that there is no return to habits of the former practice. When this goal is achieved, the change agent is removed. The change agent is the person given the task of developing and implementing the change. The final step is to evaluate the new practice to ensure it is achieving the desired goal.

Kanter (1983) describes another model of change in her book *The Change Masters*. Although Kanter suggests that change can occur at all levels of an organization, she particularly directs this model to support executives in promoting innovation and entrepreneurship in their organizations. Organizations where innovation flourishes tend to espouse a non-hierarchical structure, a team approach, consensus building as well as open and effective patterns of communication. Hence Kanter proposes three sequential 'waves of activity' reflecting innovation that supports change: problem definition, coalition building and mobilization. During problem definition, information is collected to formulate a reasonable action plan. Coalition building refers to the activities that gain support for the planned change. It requires effective communication and collaboration among organizational members. Mobilization puts the ideas into practice. Kanter espouses the need to empower employees to realize change. Therefore she recommends that leaders of innovation employ a participative approach to management. Involving appropriate stakeholders, building a team that works together, remaining receptive to the ideas of others, and sharing rewards and recognition, Kanter suggests all these processes for achieving successful innovative practice.

Health-care practices for older people are already changing and will change radically over the next few years. It is therefore urgent that health-care professionals understand the need for change and that they are proactive as leaders of change based on sound evidence. Knowledge of the types and models of change supports all health-care professionals in planning for change and responding to it. Given the current context of health and social care services, administrators and practitioners should be ready to lead the change process. Individuals who assume these roles are called change agents. It is expected that change agents view change positively and are informed about the process of change, which includes the involvement of key stakeholders, gaining support for the specific change, implementing change slowly with open lines of communication, evaluating the changed practice, and leaving the role when the change is accomplished. To be successful, administrators need to provide appropriate resources to achieve changes in practice and practitioners need to support colleagues and patients in adapting to changes in practice. Although this orientation to constant change may appear daunting at times, change is essential if health-care professionals are to remain competent, ethical and knowledgeable in keeping abreast of progress in scientific and technological advances in health and social care.

Activity

- Describe a recent change in your practice in which you apply Lewin's (1951) three-phase model of change. Specify issues that you believe should have been considered and which may have altered the implementation of the proposed change.

- Differentiate between the administrator's role and the practitioner's role in addressing a problem that requires a change in practice.
- Explain what spontaneous change means to you, someone who works in a constantly changing health-care environment. Provide examples to clarify your ideas.
- Explore the literature to identify other models of change. Reflect on the various models of change and how one of these models is applicable to your health-care setting.

KEY TRENDS INFLUENCING FUTURE HEALTH-CARE PRACTICES

Numerous factors influence the future of health-care practices today. These influences directly and indirectly affect which health-care services are provided; when, where and how professionals provide them; and ultimately, how individuals respond to health-care practices. Here are some that are tremendously influential: demography of users and providers of health-care services, epidemiology, therapeutic practices, technology, scientific discoveries such as genetic engineering and human part replacement, and the need for a multidisciplinary approach to health-care provision. They have also driven the need for changes in professional roles and responsibilities, multiprofessional working practices, promotion and development of health and social care models that promote independent partnership caring practices whereby the patient and their carers are empowered to influence the care they need.

Demography

The population is ageing (Stokes and Lindsay, 1996). This is evident from the increase in the number of individuals who are living longer, maintaining an independent lifestyle and therefore accessing health-care services for assistance in meeting home-care needs and for hospitalization during acute and chronic episodes (Miller, 1995). Basford (2001) relates the economic effect of an ageing population through its requirements for health and social care services. To reduce this economic burden, the Department of Health (2000a) proposes that health-care professionals support older people in managing their own health and lifestyle choices. Changes in health-care practices are important at a time when futurists suggest that individuals have the capacity to live longer, with the norm moving past 100 years of age. Indeed some futurists suggest that by 2050 many centenarians will be living to between 130 and 150. This view is in sharp contrast to the notion that human cells have a finite lifespan, an idea that has already been superseded, with many individuals around the world living beyond 100. This trend will definitely influence health and social care practices. Thus, governments and the populace need to address issues such as mandatory retirement, pensions and the promotion of health and well-being among older people. The promotion of healthy living throughout one's life is central to healthy living among centenarians.

Associated with longevity is the way younger populations are living their lives. For instance, the literature is replete with topics such as teenage pregnancies, fetal alcohol spectrum disorder (Abel, 1998; Cornelius *et al.*, 1997), sexually transmitted diseases, alcoholism (Chaudhuri, 2001; Dahlgren and Willander, 1989), substance abuse (Corse *et al.*, 1995) and suicides. To some degree, the future is bleak if the young of today bring to their old age the negative effects of these behaviours, effects that will undoubtedly influence the quality of their lives and whether their lives are free from disability.

Moreover, the ageing population affects the workforce in that many health-care professionals are nearing retirement or choosing to take early retirement. There is evidence to suggest this ageing workforce will result in acute shortages in many areas of practice, not only in the UK but also in the US and Canada. Clearly the shortage of nurses affects clinical practice, education and administration. This projected shortage of nurses and other health-care professionals occurs at a time when the effect of economic turbulence throughout the 1980s and 1990s resulted in downsizing, mergers and therefore losses of positions (Marquis and Huston, 2003). Simultaneously there is an increase in the demands for new nursing roles and new services. Government decisions on establishing standards of practice, funding education and promoting quality of life for health-care professionals are needed to address this significant issue if the ageing population is to be well served (Department of Health, 1999, 2000b).

Technology

There is no doubt that technology plays a critical part in all health-care services. From charting of patient information and treatment protocols to surgical procedures, technology advances the opportunities to improve health-care services. The use of technology in all facets of health care necessitates a systematic and effective information management system. Furthermore, the advances and the easy access to technological tools require that health-care professionals continue to learn how to use this new equipment and how to put the human being at the forefront of care.

Technology raises numerous issues in health-care practice. For instance, technology enables organ transplantation to happen more widely than in the past. This requires diligent attention to ethical considerations such as what organs should be used, who should receive an organ transplant, and when the organ should be made available. The ethical implications are already before many health-care teams, who have a long list of potential candidates and few organs available. Typically there are committees to address these ethical dilemmas within health-care institutions. Nonetheless, these debates are necessary if, as we expect, technology will drive the ethical dilemmas further with the effects of genetic engineering and in vitro fertilization for women in their fifties and sixties. Important questions arise: How do we provide maternal care for older women? What will be the social significance as these trends continue to strengthen? What will be the implications for children who will be teenagers when both their parents are 70 and older?

Scientific discoveries

Fortunately, researchers around the world are discovering answers to many serious health concerns. Some diseases have been eradicated, whereas others have been constrained or 'cured' by treatments. However, this success is rather short-lived. The global nature of our world is readily apparent when one reflects on severe acute respiratory syndrome (SARS) that originated in China and dramatically affected the lives of many individuals in Canada. West Nile virus has the potential to threaten lives around the world, regardless of where it originates. These diseases appear to be replicating the effects of HIV/AIDS on many populations around the globe, often decimating men and women of child-bearing years, which then leaves children orphans or nurtured by their grandparents. Furthermore, as individuals change partners, the outcomes of sexual behaviour will continue to create health-care concerns for professionals.

Taking on grandparenting roles and responsibilities is just one dimension of the equation, in that by promoting active ageing, the acceptance of divorce in old age, remarriage and the influence of drugs such as Viagra have affected the sexual behaviours of older people. Today older people are more likely to be sexually active and more likely to have multiple partners than previous older generations, so they will be at risk from sexually transmitted diseases, including HIV and AIDS. These developments challenge professional attitudes and educational needs so that health-care professionals prepare themselves to provide appropriate educational advice to older people.

Although we have considered the continued progression as a logical sequence to the advancement of old age, disease patterns do have a habit of changing. Old world diseases, such as diphtheria, poliomyelitis and tuberculosis, have not been globally eradicated; many older people would be vulnerable if an episodic outbreak or epidemic were to prevail. Unfortunately, the current education of health-care professionals does not necessarily focus on disease epidemics (new or old), so they remain relatively unprepared in preventive models or treatment regimes. The SARS incidence has highlighted this dilemma and provided useful insights to the overreaction and the unpreparedness of health-care practitioners.

Multidisciplinary approach

Unequivocally, health care is a complex and challenging business requiring professionals who can provide care from a multidimensional perspective. In this framework, health and social care professionals must be able to work together, sharing their expert knowledge and skills. Teamworking requires common understanding of each other's roles and responsibilities, and when these roles change (e.g. nurse prescribing) there is a need for each professional to provide mutual respect and support to those who have taken on these changed or extended roles. No longer is it feasible or desirable for the doctor to be the fount of all knowledge, particularly when caring for older people who have complex pathologies and social care needs. Professionals who specialize in specific areas have to develop expertise in knowledge and skill development. This expertise supports the health-care needs of individuals when they need that particular service. In institutional settings, this multidisciplinary team is readily available to meet patient needs. However, in community settings, the team is typically dispersed. Effort and commitment are needed to create opportunities for a multidisciplinary team approach to health care in many settings.

Nursing and health-care paradigm

It has been established that models of caring practice with older people have outgrown their usefulness. Care models need to engage with independent and interdependency approaches that form partnerships in care throughout the disease trajectory. There is a fixation on developments through scientific discoveries and technology but health care, particularly nursing care, is about promoting healing through a variety of modalities that do not necessarily relate to modern convention. There is a movement towards integrative health-care practice using traditional and complementary therapies, and in some fields it is happening in a most radical way. Older people are demanding these new therapeutic modes, and although laudable, it does demand an extension of the professional's knowledge base, skill and understanding. In addition, there is a need for health-care professionals to extend their knowledge and understanding of the health paradigms they currently use and to explore new hypotheses to better explain the concept of health and healing in the postmodern context.

Quantum healing as extolled by Chopra (1990) and Basford (2003) provides challenges to contemporary thinking and may stimulate debate. Similarly, Watson (2003) explains the essence of creating a caring environment, partly by reflecting on the past and present to envision a new perspective for the future. Thus, leaders consider the values, knowledge, skills and traditions on which nursing is based and resolve that the future, of necessity, needs to include this same orientation to caring and healing. Watson comments:

> To clarify and claim our deep human values and caring stance as the basis for nursing's future and past is a restoration of the heart and soul of nursing. For any profession that loses its values is soul-less; it becomes heartless and therefore becomes worthless. The worth of a profession is in clarifying, articulating, and manifesting its values

> *through action. Our values renew our energy; they inspirit our*
> *commitment and purpose for compassionate service in the world. It is*
> *our values that unite us, rather than separate. When our values are*
> *congruent with our actions, we are in harmony. We may even say we*
> *are healthy; we are whole. (ibid., p. 810)*

The pursuit of establishing new paradigms and models that reflect contemporary health care for older people requires a knowledge base that is underpinned by sound research or evidence from best practice. The Cochrane databases have exploded medical and complementary therapeutic knowledge using systematic reviews that help professionals to undertake caring practice. This service provides a synthesis of information that enables the professional workforce to keep pace with changes and the constant explosion of knowledge, thereby assuring that the professional workforces are fit and competent to practise.

The emphasis on competence is embedded in political and professional legislation. It is underpinned by the notion of continuing professional development and lifelong learning. In this climate, health-care organizations are charged with embracing the concept of learning through work and within teams (Department of Health, 2000b). This approach is a significant change in direction, in that it demands a learning culture to be implemented and resourced at every face of the organization. Learning and professional competence are no longer the sole responsibility of individuals, they become firmly cemented in organizational and personal responsibility as a joint enterprise in assuring quality of care. For example, when the scope of practice is expanded, as with nurse prescribing, it becomes the joint responsibility of the educational establishment, the organization and individuals. No longer is it acceptable that professional people adopt new roles without having the appropriate educational preparation. Nor can health-care professionals continue to practise in the modes of antiquity; they are now required to reflect critically on practice, drawing out research questions from their practice, and when appropriate, implementing research findings. Furthermore, health-care organizations must identify a research strategy that reflects local health-care needs and is in symmetry with the goals and aspirations of governments and the World Health Organization (WHO, 2002). The *National Service Framework for Older People* (Department of Health, 2001) and supporting documents reflect the research agenda for the next 10 years, but this position is likely to change as new information is disseminated from research or practice.

Educational establishments also have a responsibility to ensure that learning and teaching strategies used within their curricula facilitate the development of lifelong learning and critical reflective practice. Curricula designed to develop knowledge and skills of older people should be covered at the undergraduate and postgraduate specialist levels and should cover all elements of the lifespan throughout the programme. Learning opportunities should not focus on campus-style delivery; they should be flexible and accommodating to deliver work-related distance learning. Advancements in technology will draw on these types of learning using telemedicine and futuristic computers that do not rely on the familiar networks and resources of today. Nanotechnology has gone beyond the drawing board and is not merely the imagination of scientists.

Activity

- Identify three epidemiological factors prevalent in your area and briefly describe how these factors affect your practice.
- Describe three examples of how you use technology in your practice to promote effective care of older people.
- Explain two ethical dilemmas that have occurred within your practice in the past year.
- Explain three modern diseases that may affect older people and how your practice will be affected by these diseases.
- Describe your role in working in a multidisciplinary team.
- Explain your duty and responsibility to care for others and the significance of self-care.

LEADERSHIP SHAPING THE FUTURE OF HEALTH CARE

There is no single definition of leadership. The terms 'leader' and 'leadership' are dynamic, evoking varied definitions and theories. These theories identify characteristics, roles, functions, goals and relationships to others. Ultimately, there is the sense that we recognize leaders when we meet them and we have expectations of leaders in our work settings as well as in social and political arenas. Although leadership theories have evolved over the past 100 years, there is a call in the literature for a new kind of leadership today. This recognition that existing leadership theories do not adequately meet current needs of leadership speaks to changing environments and increasing expectations of employees and citizens.

Throughout the world there is a demand for leaders and leadership in all levels of organizations and governments to deal with the ambiguity and the challenges of providing direction to the workforce. In a Canadian example, Ginette Lemire Rodger presented an inspirational address to nurses and administrators calling for nursing leadership (Hibberd and Rodger, 1999). Rodger suggests that transformational leadership flourishes with change and innovation. She proposes four characteristics needed in nursing leaders: vision, knowledge, confidence and visibility. Vision is the ability to dream of a desired future state then to implement the needed change to achieve the goals in reality. Rodger emphasizes the need to have a vision to encourage health-care professionals to 'invest their talents, knowledge, and skills in health services' (*ibid.*, p. 262).

Rodger *ibid.* says that to realize their visions, leaders also need an effective way to employ their 'intelligence, imagination, and knowledge' (p. 263). The role of leaders in health-care sectors is complicated today because their knowledge base must extend beyond simple clinical and managerial theories and practice. Leaders in health care face an explosion of knowledge from diverse sources that directly affect service delivery: technological, economic, political, social and research. Not only do they need to know about these diverse sources, leaders also need to understand how to anticipate and respond to their influences. Moreover, leaders need to consider their employees and support the development of knowledge work teams within learning organizations (Senge, 1990).

Rodger also highlights the importance of confidence if leaders are to orchestrate change amid uncertainty. Health-care leaders are deemed credible when they demonstrate self-confidence and knowledge about issues, possible solutions and potential responses to various decisions. Leaders also demonstrate their self-esteem when they confront difficult situations head-on and with enthusiasm. Moreover, visibility of leaders is critical if they are to support professional roles and to have a voice in decision-making processes. Speaking about the imperative for nursing leadership, Rodger states, 'We need nursing leaders who are proud to be nurses, but who are effective and visible while creating partnerships in the delivery of an integrated healthcare service' (Hibberd and Rodger, 1999, p. 265). The four characteristics – vision, knowledge, confidence and visibility – prepare leaders to effect change to foster quality standards in providing health and social services.

Porter-O'Grady (2000) comments: 'In less than sixty years the entire landscape for health service has been so radically altered that it has transformed all members of society' (p. 31). In this new age, health-care professionals and patients remain uncertain about what to expect from change and how to respond to it. Without doubt, leaders are integral players who need to be future oriented, poised to move forward into the unknown without glancing back to retain former practices. Leaders need to envision a changed and improved future state and lead others to realize the need for a fundamentally different modus operandi. Porter-O'Grady captures the essence of this requirement when he states:

> *The work of leadership is not assuring that the staff can survive the current chaos in health service. It is instead about designing new ways of working and living in a paradigm for health service that bears little resemblance to that into which most of us began the work of our professions. (ibid., p. 32)*

As the future continues to evolve, Porter-O'Grady suggests that thriving in this new age requires 'doing and being different' (*ibid.*, p. 32). He notes the ageing cohort of baby boomers and suggests that health and social services will be hard pressed to meet the demands of this population unless there are significant changes in service. He concludes, 'The agenda for leadership is how it will create the demand and conditions for confronting the conflict between professional attachment to past practice and the growing demand for a different context and content for health services' (*ibid.*, p. 37). The leader is charged with a daunting task not only of reading the future but of creating the conditions for essential change.

Leaders invest their tremendous talents in moving organizations forward to realize goals and ensure quality standards are achieved. However, it is abundantly clear that leaders do not achieve their visions independently; they require a team of professionals who can enact those quality standards in a multitude of settings.

Activity

- Describe the evolution of leadership theories. This information is readily available in many nursing and general management texts.
- Identify six key differences between leaders and managers.
- Discuss whether leadership is an innate ability or a developed ability.
- Identify a leader within your area of practice and discuss why you think they are providing leadership.
- Differentiate between transformational and transactional leadership. Refer to Burns (1978) and current literature for discussions on these types of leadership.

RESEARCH STRATEGIES OF THE DEPARTMENT OF HEALTH

Evidence-based practice is now expected of all health-care professionals. Significantly the global research community readily shares findings to support the advancement of knowledge and practice. Ultimately, the goal is to provide individuals with quality health and social care in all settings around the world. No nation should be deprived of health-care services, although many developing countries continue to function with basic medical provision. Nevertheless, the advances gleaned through research into how practice might change have the potential to support citizens of all countries. Through the Cochrane Library, it is possible to obtain up-to-date information on treatments and results. Access to the literature is only the first step in realizing a change in practice. Health-care professionals should apply their critical-thinking skills in reviewing this literature and determining whether or not to change practice in their setting. Health-care professionals have an obligation to remain current with the best practice and to ensure they are competent and caring practitioners.

In 2002 the World Health Organization produced a document outlining a policy framework for active ageing. This document was timely, given the attention to this topic in the UK and around the world. For instance, over the past decade, the Department of Health produced numerous documents focusing on older people. These documents provide background data to support the ageing population by identifying specific needs of this group (Department of Health, 2001), promoting strategies and programmes to improve services (Department of Health, 2002b), and establishing standards of care (Department of Health, 2000a).

SUMMARY

The future of health-care services was discussed from the perspectives of trends, change, leadership and their effect on older people. Numerous trends are evident that directly affect the opportunities and challenges within health care. For instance, advances in technology have created the opportunity to transplant organs and this has led to ethical challenges in determining who should receive those organs. These trends create a health-care sector in a constant state of flux. Three types of change were briefly described: developmental change, spontaneous change and planned change. Two models of change were discussed. Leaders in health-care organizations are instrumental in visualizing a changed future. Moreover, they play key roles in assisting practitioners to embrace changes in practice with enthusiasm and competence. Ultimately, all health-care professionals are obliged to engage in lifelong learning so that quality standards in health and social care are maintained. Our patients deserve the best care we can provide, and only when all members of the multidisciplinary team work together can we realize the essence of professional practice that improves quality of care in a seamless and effective manner.

Key points ▶

1 Change is constant in all spheres of life.
2 Trends in demography, scientific discovery, medical advances and technology have dramatic effects on health and social care services.
3 These trends determine the best treatments available for older people, taking into account that the population is ageing.
4 Theoretical models exist to ensure success from the challenging but rewarding change process.
5 The change process is typically initiated by a change agent, who is expected to lead the process and often leaves the organization when the change has been implemented and adopted by employees.
6 Leaders are needed at all levels of a health-care organization.
7 The definitions of 'leader' and 'leadership' remain elusive, but individuals tend to recognize a leader and the effect of leadership.
8 To be effective, leaders need to be visionary, knowledgeable, confident and visible.

9 Knowledge of the past informs the present and the future of health and social care services.

10 When governments respond to changing environments with sound policy and resources, the results can have positive effects on the citizens.

REFERENCES

Abel, E. L. (1998) Protecting fetuses from certain harm. *Politics and the Life Sciences*, **17**(2), 113–117.

Basford, L. (2001) Quantum healing: nursing therapy [president's column, e-nursing]. *Journal of the European Honours Society for Nurses and Midwives*, **1**(1), 1–3.

Basford, L. (2003) Complementary therapies. In: *Theory and Practice of Nursing: An Integrated Approach to Caring Practice*, 2nd edn (ed. Basford, L. and Slevin, O.). Nelson Thornes, Cheltenham, Glos., pp. 569–596.

Chaudhuri, J. D. (2001) Prenatal alcohol exposure: a review. *Frontiers in Fetal Health*, **3**(4), 107–114.

Chopra, D. (1990) *Quantum Healing: Exploring the Frontiers of Mind/Body Medicine*. Bantum, London.

Cornelius, M. D., Lebow, H. A. and Day, N. L. (1997) Attitudes and knowledge about drinking: relationships with drinking behavior among pregnant teenagers. *Journal of Drug Education*, **27**(3), 231–243.

Corse, S. J., McHugh, M. K. and Gordon, S. M. (1995) Enhancing provider effectiveness in treating pregnant women with addictions. *Journal of Substance Abuse Treatment*, **12**(1), 3–12.

Dahlgren, L. and Willander, A. (1989) Are special treatment facilities for female alcoholics needed? A controlled 2-year follow-up study from a specialized female unit (EWA) versus a mixed male/female treatment facility. *Alcoholism: Clinical and Experimental Research*, **13**(4), 499–504.

Department of Health (1999) *Making a Difference: Strengthening the Nursing, Midwifery and Health Visiting Contribution to Health and Health Care*. The Stationery Office, London.

Department of Health (2000a) *Care Homes for Older People: National Minimum Standards*. The Stationery Office, London.

Department of Health (2000b) *The National Health Service Ten-Year Plan*. The Stationery Office, London.

Department of Health (2001) *National Service Framework for Older People*. The Stationery Office, London.

Department of Health (2002a) *The Care Standards Act 2000: A Guide for Registered Service Providers*. The Stationery Office, London.

Department of Health (2002b) *Information Strategy for Older People in England*. The Stationery Office, London.

Hibberd, J. M. and Rodger, G. L. (1999) Contemporary perspectives on leadership. In: *Nursing Management in Canada*, 2nd edn (ed. Hibberd, J. M. and Smith, D. L.). W. B. Saunders, Toronto, pp. 259–277.

Kanter, R. M. (1983) *The Change Masters: Innovation and Entrepreneurship in the American Corporation*. Touchstone, New York.

Lewin, K. (1951) *Field Theory in Social Science*. Harper & Row, New York.

Marquis, B. L. and Huston, C. J. (2003) *Leadership Roles and Management Functions in Nursing Theory and Application*, 4th edn. Lippincott, Philadelphia PA.

Miller, J. F. (1995) Four nurses enhance elderly care. *Reflections*, **21**(3), 9–10.

Porter-O'Grady, T. (2000) Visions for the 21st century: new horizons, new health care. *Nursing Administration Quarterly*, **25**(1), 30–38.

Senge, P. M. (1990) *The Fifth Discipline: The Art and Practice of the Learning Organization*. Doubleday, New York.

Skelton-Green, J. (1999) Managing change. In: *Nursing Management in Canada*, 2nd edn (ed. Hibberd, J. M. and Smith, D. L.). W. B. Saunders, Toronto, pp. 455–479.

Stokes, J. and Lindsay, J. (1996) Major causes of death and hospitalisation in Canadian seniors. *Chronic Diseases in Canada*, **17**(2), 63–73.

Watson, J. (2003) Into the future: post-modern and beyond. In: *Theory and Practice of Nursing: An Integrated Approach to Caring Practice*, 2nd edn (ed. Basford, L. and Slevin, O.). Nelson Thornes, Cheltenham, Glos., pp. 808–811.

WHO (2002) *Active Ageing: A Policy Framework*. World Health Organization, Geneva.

FURTHER READING

Burns, J. M. (1978) *Leadership*. Harper & Row, New York.

Appendix: Mary and Heather

Mary's experience

Mary's medical history
- **1989**: heart operation for an aneurysm
- **1993**: broken leg
- **Nov 1996**: fall; discharged from accident and emergency
- **Nov/Dec 1996**: hip replacement operation
- **Dec 1996**: suspected clot on lung, and pneumonia
- **Dec 1996**: deep-vein thrombosis
- **Mar 1997**: referral to day hospital

Introduction
Mary is 70 years old. Her husband, who had been in the army, died several years ago. At one time, his army work meant frequent moves to different localities, which has meant that Mary has lived in 30 different houses during her lifetime. She has lived in her present council house for 20 years.

Mary has six children: three sons and three daughters. Her sons are married with families and live outside London. Her youngest daughter (aged 36 years) is Heather. Heather and her husband, Ron, and their children Emily (aged 10) and Tommy (aged 4) live with Mary. Mary's eldest daughter, Sandra, lives with her family on the other side of London. Her middle daughter, Caroline, lives with her family in the Midlands.

Mary's narrative traces her health history over the past decade. She talks of her experiences of a heart operation and a broken leg and more recent experiences of a hip replacement and a suspected clot on her lungs which turned out to be pneumonia. Her most recent experience of hospital is that following a deep-vein thrombosis and referral to a day hospital. The rest of this section is in Mary's own words and the next section is in Heather's own words.

The family
Heather goes out to work. She has two children. Whoever gets in first does the cooking – it's usually me four days a week. Sometimes you can get the children to help but the four-year-old, well, he's just an ordinary four-year-old.

We've got three rooms downstairs, the lounge and the dining room leading to the kitchen, and a small toilet. Upstairs there are the bedrooms and the bathroom.

Work

I have a small part-time job, bookkeeping three days a week. I have to get two buses. I enjoy my work. They say I'll be able to manage again but we'll have to see.

I do like my work. I enjoy it. I've done some at home, actually, since I've been back out of hospital, but I would like to go back. I work three times a week so it's not too hectic, you know. Usually I do Monday, Wednesday and Friday, which is just right. If there's something more that wants doing on a Tuesday then I'll change my days. You know, it's fairly flexible. I can really do the three days when I want to do them, so it's quite good, actually.

The heart operation

I've got no complaints about the treatments I've had, or anything, because I think they're excellent. My children don't like the hospital, they think it's a terrible place. My oldest daughter is a bit prejudiced, actually. Well, I went in to have a heart op, bypass, because I had an aneurysm and they wouldn't touch the aneurysm until they'd done my heart. For some unknown reason the doctors don't know, I didn't come round for two days. I had the op done on the Thursday and by the time I sort of came round it turned out to be late Saturday night. I thought it was still Thursday. I remember seeing my son and daughter-in-law and didn't know what day it was. It was Sunday before I really came round and then I got confused a couple of times.

Evidently, while I was, I don't know whether you'd call it unconscious or what, but while I wasn't with it, my daughter had phoned up and they said I was having physiotherapy. Well, when she came in I was still out, so of course she hit the roof.

The doctor said to her: 'Well, your mother's very diseased, she's got very diseased arteries,' and she said: 'Well, why did you tell me that she was having physio?' I said: 'I could have been having physio for all you know'; it is quite possible because I've seen it happen on the ward. But as I say, this doctor or whoever he was, I don't know who he was, he definitely put her off the hospital.

The broken leg

I don't know, but I broke that leg. I'd only stepped across the road and fell over. I tripped and went flying. The physio came here; she came here twice a week to give me exercises when I got out of plaster. I was in plaster for three months and she thought I'd torn my tendon at the back.

The broken hip

Whether I've damaged it [the leg] again I don't know. I think I may have done when I fell.

I was at the top of the stairs and I turned to come down – I was more or less coming down backwards and I missed my footing and that's when I went flying.

My son complained first of all about the fact that I fell the week before I had my operation. I went in the day I fell because the pain had got so bad – I'd gone to bed, actually. I went into casualty and they were quite convinced that all I'd done was torn a muscle or bruised a muscle, or what have you. I didn't get an X-ray and they sent me home. I was wandering around on the crutches and it gradually got worse. By the following weekend the pain was absolutely unbearable and I was in tears and that was when I got the doctor and she thought I'd done the femur and she said they'd pin it.

Well, I went back in that day; she got an ambulance and they were still saying I hadn't broken anything and that was why he started to complain. Eventually they did an X-ray and found out the head was damaged so I had it done the following day. Then I lost a tooth! The poor doctor was very apologetic; she gave it to me in a little pot. She said: 'It got very wobbly.' Well, I knew it was wobbly. I knew a couple of my front teeth were wobbly so it didn't really surprise me. Mind you, I'm feeling a bit of a jack now! No point complaining about that.

I said to Heather: 'Well, that's it; I'm not having any more operations.' She said: 'Why not?' I said: 'Because every time I have one something happens and I end up in and out of hospital for weeks.' But I suppose it's just one of those things.

That was the reason my son complained – because I got discharged, but I honestly think that that could have been my fault because as far as I was concerned that was where the pain was; that was where it hurt me. It still hurts a bit but it's not like it was then. I fell on my back, I mean the bottom of my spine really hurt that day, and I told them that and I think that's where probably some of the confusion lay. I could only tell them where it hurt me. I think I must have pulled something because it's still bad, not as bad as it was – sometimes it's worse than others. Perhaps I'm trying to get around too much; I do too much or stand up too long.

I think sometimes you tend to blot out things; you don't want to sort of bother anybody with little things. I don't know about anybody else, but I feel sometimes that I haven't been quite honest with them as to what I can do and what I can't do. You can't blame them; it's your own fault.

They made certain that I'd got gadgets that help me, and so forth, but if I hadn't said anything they probably wouldn't have. I'm not saying they wouldn't have bothered but I mean it would in a sense have been my own fault. I mean, if you don't tell anybody they're not going to know, are they?

So in a sense I would consider it half my fault if they don't give me the information I need, and sometimes when you've been in and out of hospital you're in such a hurry to get home and fed up with being in the hospital that you forget all the things you should ask.

The only thing that got me was that I can't hear very well. I can't always hear correctly. But all the doctors that I saw were very good at explaining and telling me what they were going to do, and what have you. I've no complaints at all. I'm not very good at explaining things myself. I think sometimes I could unconsciously have given them the wrong impression. That was probably why I never had it done in the first place. As far as I was concerned that was where it hurt. I'm not very good at explaining things, I know that, and I could have given them the wrong impression and also got the wrong impression, too, because I can't hear very well. I think it's 50/50 sometimes – more 100% on my part than theirs.

I still try to do the exercises they tell me to do with the hip; it is very difficult and it does hurt sometimes. I do try; admittedly I don't do them as often as I should. She said I should do it ten times. I can't always do it so I do two or three when I first stand up, perhaps on the crutches, you know, after I want to get up to go to the toilet or something, but I don't do ten all at once – I just can't. I do try and do some at least during the day; it's only a couple of small exercises, one sort of lifting the leg and then another one. She said it was like ballet dancing. There were two of us and she said: 'You can do them together.'

Suspected clot on lung/pneumonia

I think it was about ten o'clock at night; the nurse who admitted me was very good. Sadly, I never saw her again, there was always a different lot on but she was very, very good, very concerned as well. She did care and she made certain she knew what had happened and that sort of thing. At that time of night I think the poor old night staff always seem to get the worst of it, but she was very good.

She was concerned with how I was and she asked my daughter quite a lot of questions, and so forth. She made sure I was fairly comfortable and she did ask if I wanted a hot drink. She made sure I had water, and what have you. She wasn't the sort who chucks you in the bed. She did stay with me and she asked Heather questions, too.

As far as I'm concerned, the admitting staff have always been very good; they've never just sort of admitted you and then tucked you up in bed. If they think you're a bit depressed or something they sort of make certain they stay with you for a little while, get you a drink or whatever you might need. I have found that they've always been very good once I've got to the wards.

It was difficult to talk to the nurses because there was never very many of them; it was a big ward and I sometimes felt sorry for the poor staff. How they coped with all of us I don't know – we were all different; some were bedridden. They were good although they were rushed off their feet; they didn't have the staff, and the staff levels were terrible. It was the same on the other ward – the fracture ward – sometimes there were only three on for twenty-odd beds. That's not many, not a great lot of staff. It was a large ward, and mixed as well, which couldn't have helped matters. Apart from that I found the staff quite helpful, and if they had had the time to stop and talk they would have; they didn't, but it wasn't always possible for them to.

They explained about the clot on the lung. I will give him [the doctor] his due: when I had the final scan he came up within an hour and explained that everything was all right, there was no clot – there were no problems – and I thought that was very good; it relieved my mind. He came and told me that the results were clear and what I had was probably pneumonia. He said they can't always differentiate between pneumonia and a clot on the lung, which is fair enough. I don't expect miracles from anybody because none of us can perform them. Then he said I could go home the next day and I was very pleased. Mind you, I didn't expect to be back in another three days.

Transport home

You know the awful thing about when I was sat in the reception for two hours waiting for transport after the pneumonia. I was just stuck there in the wheelchair and I couldn't do anything. There was a girl at the help desk and she was no help, either. I mean she must have known I was sat there for a couple of hours. All they sent was a cab. The cab driver came and asked me who I was, you know, asked me if I was Mary Fisher. I said yes and he said: 'I've come to take you,' and I said: 'Well, I can't walk to a cab.' He looked at me and he said: 'You can't walk?' I said: 'No, I can't,' so of course he went. I mean, it wasn't his job to take me to the cab in a wheelchair anyway.

I'd been there about half an hour, I think, and then I was sat there for the next I don't know how long. Luckily, I saw a friend of mine who lives in the next road and she stayed with me and they finally got my son-in-law. He was most annoyed. He'd been home since 6.00 p.m. and he could have come and got me and been done with it. He was absolutely fuming; he wasn't very pleased at all because nobody knew where I was. My daughters had rung up the ward and found out that they'd already taken me out of the ward and as far as they knew, as far as the ward was concerned, I'd gone home. I was still in the hospital; I mean, I can see the funny side of it afterwards, but I didn't see the funny side when I was sat there. One of the nurses came down and she was very concerned. Why on earth didn't the girl on the help desk come over and speak to me? I shouted to her three or four times, but she took no notice. She sort of looked at me. There was nobody else there; it's the first time it's ever happened. I hope it never happens again. I thought I was there for ever. Mind you, my son's complained since; he's written a few letters to the hospital. I didn't know until last week. I mean they have replied to them; I'll give them their due. I got a letter of apology about being left there.

When I was discharged [after the deep-vein thrombosis] my son-in-law decided he wasn't having any more of me sitting around for two hours, so he came and fetched me. I had two of them actually, two sons-in-law and they were very good. When they got here they carried me out, picked me up between them and carried me back indoors. I had a frame which was supposed to go back to the hospital and the girls brought that out so that I could get indoors with the frame, but the boys decided just to carry me – good job I trusted them.

No, nobody from the hospital has ever travelled with me, unless I've been in an ambulance – one of those small ambulances. Well, it didn't particularly worry me, as long as I got home and I could manage to get out of the car and indoors.

I was under the impression when I was discharged that they'd arranged all the transport; I was under the impression that it was hospital transport, not a cab. I'd been stuck in bed for a couple of days so I was having to get mobile again. The care I had I was quite content with, I suppose. It was just bad luck as regards sort of sitting around waiting for transport to take me home – it was just one of those things. The kids weren't very pleased, but they're never pleased with anything, anyway, so what's the difference?

Deep-vein thrombosis

Post-discharge
I've not been too bad except for the leg – it started this afternoon: it is a bit swollen around the knee. Probably I should walk around a bit more. It only started today. I'll see what it is like tomorrow; if it is still as bad I'll get my GP in. It doesn't feel too bad; maybe it is because I've got it up. I don't want to go back to hospital; I've been in twice this time.

The knee is a bit blue. It seems to be going down, though; probably because I've got it up a bit higher now it doesn't look quite so blue. Eventually it will all go down, I hope. Actually it has gone down; it is not as slim as that one – well that is skinny – but it has gone down; you can see the knee now.

Five or six days later
Five or six days later my leg was swollen; as one of my daughters put it, it was like a tree trunk. So we got the GP and I went back into hospital, this time with a thrombosis. Well, they didn't know if I'd get home for Christmas or not but I did come home – on Christmas eve, actually. By that time they'd put me on warfarin and everything else and that was it. But I still wasn't convinced. My leg was very painful at the top. I could walk – I had a frame – but that was just about all.

Outpatients
I have to go back next Thursday for a hospital appointment but it's at another hospital. Why, I don't know. It's a medical clinic so I presume it's for the pneumonia. I don't see what else it can be because if it was my hip it would be the fracture clinic. The only thing I can think of is the lung. Anyway, they're sending transport because otherwise I couldn't get there.

I had a clinic appointment for the fracture clinic while I was in but they took me down from the ward. They were very good, actually, and I wasn't down there very long. When I broke my leg I sat there for hours before I saw anyone. I saw them quite quickly – I was down in the clinic at quarter past nine and I was back upstairs in the ward by ten o'clock, which to me is very good.

Day hospital

I think it's a lovely hospital, the staff at the day hospital are really, really good. It doesn't matter what you say. We have a nice lunch as well. No, they do look after you. Oh, I think they're gorgeous [the staff at day hospital], they're really friendly. They'll have a laugh and a joke with you and it's not like an ordinary hospital.

They sent me to the day hospital. She [the doctor] said: 'I think we ought to get some physio for you and arrange for you to go to the day hospital.'

I hadn't a clue what the day hospital was. I've been attending since March and I was just getting back nicely until a few weeks ago when I fell in the hospital. I don't know what happened but I just lost my balance. I couldn't stop myself and I went flying. They were very good, they've been excellent at the day hospital, really they have. Luckily I hadn't done any damage, but they sent me straight down to the X-ray department and X-rayed everything just to make sure I was okay. It took me back onto two sticks. Somebody asked me, I think it was the physio, if I wanted my crutches back. I told her: 'No, thank you very much.' She laughed. I've just managed over the past couple of days to go onto one stick again, except when I went out. I'd be scared to use one stick to go out but I'm on one stick indoors so I'm quite pleased with myself and I can get up and down the stairs.

I went to the day hospital twice a week when they finally rang me, and I had a letter confirming that they would pick me up on the Monday. I went on a Monday and a Thursday and then I was supposed to get discharged but I fell over being clumsy. I've only been going once a week since. Hopefully I should get discharged in about two weeks' time, well, she said so – unless anything else happens.

Usually I'm in there by 11; well, it depends what time the ambulance gets here to pick me up. I mean, sometimes we can be there very early but it's not very often. I usually get there between ten and eleven and they're very good. You get your blood pressure and everything else taken first and a cup of tea or whatever you want. Then you more or less sit around until lunchtime, unless of course you've got X-rays or something, but they're usually done after lunch. Sometimes the physio gets there before lunchtime, but not always.

When I first started attending they used to wheel me down to the gym and give me exercises on the bed and then eventually I graduated and was able to walk. I've been out in the grounds for a walk when it's nice and I'm very pleased actually because at least my leg is mobile. It still hurts sometimes; some days it's worse than others. If I sit too long it gets a bit swollen, that's why I put it up. Somebody said it was the heat and then I went back to my doctor and he said it was the intense cold, so I give up on that one.

They give us lunch at the day hospital, and then blood tests. The first day is murder because you've got everything – blood tests, X-rays; you name it, they do it. Then if they think you need X-rays in between you go. I went down last Monday for one – they decided to X-ray the spine. In between they arranged for me to go to the osteoporosis clinic where they found I have got osteoporosis. Probably that's why I keep fracturing things. I never broke anything until three years ago when I broke my leg.

They said that they would give me physio there. The doctor said she thought twice a week would be better for me but they weren't certain how the day hospital could fit it in. I had to wait until I went there and then they decided that I would go twice a week. I went regularly then on Mondays and Thursdays. The ambulance picked me up every time and there was never any problem with that, and if I had another appointment at the hospital then they arranged transport for that for me as well, so they're very, very good.

We usually read the papers and we have a chat between us because there's quite a few go there; you get to know people eventually who go on the same days as you and you end up sort of getting friendly with them and it's quite nice, actually. The staff are absolutely wonderful: there's only three nurses and a care assistant and they're absolutely run off their feet sometimes because they do everything. There's a doctor as well and he's lovely; it really is friendly there.

People don't want to be discharged from the day hospital. You get to know everybody.

HEATHER'S EXPERIENCE

Background

I was 16 when we moved here and then I met my husband and we decided to stay here because I didn't like to leave Mum on her own, although she was much younger then. It's a council property. We've only been married for ten years. Mum would have been here by herself because by that time all my brothers and sisters had gone and left. We were all very young when we got the house; it would have meant that maybe Mum would have had to give it up for a smaller place, and she's moved about 30 times in her life.

Well, my Dad was in the forces so she followed him wherever he went – I think that we'd been living here for so long that she didn't want to move. It was handy for us really; we've got our own bit upstairs – we've got our own space. We've got a front room upstairs as well. So we've been living here all this time. We've got no plans to move; this is Mum's house really, not ours. We've been here for a long time.

I've always lived here and I've never left. I think that my husband decided that I wasn't going anywhere so he'd have to come here and it's not as though the house is small; it's fine. I'm sure my children get on Mum's nerves sometimes; she's always had children around her, you see, so I'm sure she'd like a bit of peace, but we do leave her alone a lot. It's basically like having two flats, except that we use the same kitchen and the same bathroom, although not at the moment.

It is nice; I mean I wouldn't dream of going now, especially now Mum's not well, but I don't want to go so I'm quite happy to stay here and the children are happy here. I mean if we were to move, if we were to be rehoused by the council, we'd probably get a flat, and at the moment we've got a nice garden, a nice big house: the children have each got a bedroom. It's fine for us. They would have to move Mum as well, and I think she'd be very, very unhappy if she had to move. She's always said: 'I wouldn't mind living by myself,' but she doesn't want to move, I know that. We moved in here, she didn't move in with us.

Am I a carer? I'm just her daughter, I've never classed myself as a carer before. In some ways I feel it's my duty; I mean, I couldn't just go off and leave her. In the mornings she's not been able to get to the sink because her leg's been painful so we have to get a bowl of water and towels and her soap and everything, so everything's basically brought to her.

It doesn't bother me; sometimes I get tired, sometimes I get fed up, but I've also got two young children to run around after in the morning and they get on my nerves more. It's just hard. Ideally, I'd like to be here; I'd like to be able to maybe work less hours so that I could be here and just take it all in my stride. I also feel it puts pressure on Mum sometimes because in a way I feel I'm rushing her. In the morning, as I say, I have to get up, so that means Mum has to get up at a certain time and do these things in a certain time before I leave for work. It's not a burden; it's a strain. I think also she feels that she's putting pressure on me and I'm sure it must get her down as well, for someone who's been so active, I mean. She did go to work before all this happened. I'm sure it's harder for her than it is for me.

She was working three days a week and it was hard for her; the other two days she'd spend at home. When I came home there was a meal cooked because she was still able to do all those things – she came back so quickly when she broke her leg. This one has just put her completely out so I think she must think about how she's going to be in the future.

Last November she had a fall down the stairs and she couldn't walk very well afterwards. She was taken into the hospital and they sent her home with some painkillers. She couldn't take the pain so she went back in and they found that she'd broken her hip. She had a hip replacement, came home and then she got a thrombosis. No, no, she got pneumonia first and she was taken back for a week, then she came home for a few days and then she got a thrombosis in her leg, so she was taken back. She came home on Christmas eve last year; well, she just sat in a corner and dozed off most of the time. She wasn't able to get around for another few weeks and obviously she became weak.

Yes, she was working; she's not gone back and she's not going to. I think she's quite got used to the fact now.

Experience of the hospital

There were times when we telephoned to see how she was, to ask if they wanted her frame brought in and if she was supposed to get out of bed. They'd say things like: 'Well, if she wants to, she can,' and I thought that was a bit strange because of the hip replacement. She'd only been home a week, so obviously she was still very immobile. It kind of made us a bit confused as to whether they were aware of why she got the pneumonia in the first place and basically how to deal with it.

I tell you another thing that I was a bit concerned about: they'd get her out of bed and sit her in the chair but they never came back and asked if she was all right; she had to attract their attention.

There was an incident just after she had the hip replacement: the nurse laid her on her side, the bad side, and left her all night. I can't remember if it was the time when the buzzer on her bed wasn't working so she couldn't call them; I don't know if that was that time. I don't want it to sound as though I'm complaining all the time, but I think there are certain things that can be looked at. The next morning, because she hadn't slept very well on her bad side, she was really down and from what I gather she had a go at the nurse and upset the nurse. 'Tough,' I said. I know they're busy, I can see they're busy, I see it when I go there and I see them racing around. If you've got a ward full of elderly people who can't care for themselves it's hard; I know there have been cutbacks and it's sad because there's no time for the patients anymore. I've sat in wards and I've seen elderly people who can't feed themselves and there's no one there to feed them. When she had the thrombosis, the ward seemed a bit more caring but it was a smaller ward. Some of those big wards are quite scary. You think: 'Oh, gosh, I have to go home and leave her here.' It's a big shame.

In the ward at the hospital they have a certain nurse taking care of whatever area your bed is in. When I spoke to them they didn't seem to know much; you'd ask how she was and they'd say: 'Oh, she's fine; she's had her breakfast and she's sitting up,' and that's it. But we knew she was sitting up anyway; she couldn't lie down because of the pain in her chest. We just thought: 'They must know what they're talking about.'

No, no we never got a named nurse. I don't know if they used agency nurses in there; they changed shifts a lot: when she was first admitted we were given a card with a name on it, but I never saw that nurse again or spoke to her. I think I can remember her telling me that wasn't her ward, anyway, she was only there covering, so I don't know.

I suppose you could have spoken to the nurses, but it was very rare that we saw a doctor and it was very difficult to be able to speak to a doctor. Obviously when you're there they have to page him – he might be in an emergency, he might be doing this, he might be doing that, so that was really, really difficult.

I probably wouldn't have asked anybody, but I wouldn't even have known who to ask. Do you ask the nurses or do you ask the doctor when and if you can see them?

There are lots of things that have made us a bit cross with the hospital, I mean the fact that she was sent home in the first place with a broken hip when she first fell; then when she was left in the corridor for the two hours. The quicker she came out of the place the better we felt, although it was hard. We're not nurses; we only do the best we can and if something's wrong we don't know what to do.

Preparation for home

I was always scared. We never knew if she was definitely coming home. They'd say the previous day: 'Oh, you might be able to go home tomorrow,' and then you'd have to phone the hospital because you think: 'Oh, yeah, we'll have to find out,' and then we'd phone and then maybe they'd tell us: 'Well, we're not sure yet,' and then a few hours later we'd phone back and they'd say: 'Yes, she's allowed home.' How do you prepare? I wouldn't know how to prepare. I wouldn't know what she's capable of doing, what she should be doing, what she shouldn't be doing after she's had an operation. I mean, I don't know.

Transport home

The night she was left waiting in the corridor she was so glad to be home. The woman on the help desk got a bit of a mouthful from my husband – he wasn't very happy.

It hits you personally. I thought: 'Oh Mum, you want affection really.' I mean, we'd all like affection. We'd want them taken home in an ambulance, carried in if they can't walk. We know that's not possible, but I think there are steps that could be taken to help.

At home after discharge

I was a bit concerned when she came home because to me she didn't seem well. We have a toilet down here but she still had to use the four steps down. We practically had to beg for a commode, because they felt that she should be getting about on her leg: if they gave her one they felt that she might just depend on that. That wasn't the case: she wasn't well and it was difficult for her. She did actually fall not long after she came out from having the pneumonia; she fell again coming down the stairs – that was before they put the bars in.

She doesn't use the commode anymore – there's a toilet in the bathroom upstairs, which is on the same landing as her bedroom, and during the day she uses the one behind the kitchen.

She used the commode when she was sleeping downstairs.

When she had the bad diarrhoea I used the toilet frame with the bucket, so it was a bit distressful for Mum. It didn't bother me at all, but it was distressful for Mum.

Social services

Because it said in her notes that she lived with her daughter and son-in-law they may think socially at home she's fine, but there are certain things in the house, like layout. I mean, she's got to be able to go to the toilet; she's got to come down the stairs. She's not very good; she's fallen since. Okay, it wasn't a drastic fall, but it could have been if no one had been here; it happened in the evening. Luckily, I was here.

Working

I'm here full-time. I'm here, I live here, but I have to work as well. We both have to go to work, and we work full-time, and during the day it's worrying. The only thing I can do is phone up, and if the phone isn't answered and I try again and it's still not answered, I rush home. When she first came home there was an incident where she wasn't answering the phone and I tried again twenty minutes later. She still didn't answer the phone and I came rushing home because I had visions of her having fallen.

Unfortunately, when she was in hospital it was the busiest period at work, because I work in retail and it was Christmas time. You think to yourself: 'Oh my God, I have to go into work and tell them I have to go home.' They're really very good about it, but in a way you're thinking: 'Well, I don't want to overstep the mark.' Do you see what I mean? I mean, it may not sound very nice and very caring, but it's trying to draw the line between which one is your main priority. At the end of the day you've still got to work: you've still got to bring home money to feed your family and, unfortunately, we don't get any help, so it was very difficult.

I'd say they are sympathetic at work – they are to you, but you don't know what they're saying behind your back. Like I said, you don't know what your main priority is – you don't want it to seem like you're taking advantage.

Caring

You read about staff cuts in the newspapers and everything and you can see it's for real. That's why we'd rather have her home and care for her here – we'd like to care for her better than we do, we'd like to know that we're caring for her properly, but we try to do what's best. I try not to do too much because I don't want to be told off by Mum. The worst thing is that, even now, at this age, you're scared of your Mum telling you off.

I think it might have been helpful to have been able to be around when she had the therapist in hospital: when she first came home and she had to manage the stairs I didn't have a clue. Should I stand behind her, do I stand in front of her, do I help her down, do I just leave her alone and let her come down on her own or should I watch that she's doing it right? You know, those sorts of things. I would have liked to have been at home for the whole time. Okay, maybe not when Mum was in hospital because I'd be sitting at home, but when she came home it would have been ideal.

There are certain things I would have liked to have seen: what the therapist was doing with her and how she did it, so that I could be more help when she came home. I don't know if I get on Mum's nerves, maybe I'm a hindrance – I'm there always behind her when she's coming down the stairs, I might make her nervous, it's very difficult to know. It's like helping her up and down the stairs – you think to yourself maybe you should have found out if you should help her, or just let her get on with it. I mean, for all I know, she could be coming down the stairs fine, it's the way the picture shows on the chart they gave us, but to me the way she's coming down looks a bit dangerous and it's ever so painful. I try not to fuss too much or else I get told off. I'd rather worry silently than fuss because I get told off and I can't bear that – it's no different from when you're a little girl, it still feels the same.

Obviously I have to work all day. I used to do her lunch for her, or come home from work and do lunch, but now she can manage all that for herself, and her breakfast. She can manage to cook but she wouldn't be able to get heavy things out of the oven or out of the fridge; she's fine with basic things. If I was late for any reason she'd have cooked the potatoes and things like that; it's just heavy things that she can't really lift. If I put a chicken in the oven she wouldn't be able to lift it out, but simple things on top of the stove she's fine with. It doesn't really matter about things like the housework, washing and ironing, because we're here, so I do that anyway.

The GP, district nurse and warfarin

At first we were very worried because she has to take the warfarin now because of the thrombosis, and it was getting her down. She'd have to go to the hospital every week or every other week or twice a week to have blood tests, but luckily enough we've got a good GP and she sorted that out. I don't know if she told you, the district nurse is coming in, so that's good. That was a worry. There were lots of little worries we had. I think we would have had them anyway – I mean, Mum's not getting any younger, so we worry anyway.

The GP was more than happy to be able to send the nurse and get it done at home, and it seems to have worked well. It certainly cheered Mum up when she heard – she was over the moon, really.

I think I trust more in the GP than in the hospital – not being rude – but you know, after the trouble she had I think it makes you a bit wary and the GP's been really good. The hospital was very surprised when the GP agreed to get the district nurse to come out and do the blood tests because they thought that there was no way they would do it, but she's very good, and she knows what Mum's been through.

The day hospital

The day hospital are definitely planning to get her mobile again and to do some pain control. How they do that I don't know.

I'm just dreading the first time she goes to the day hospital, because of the newness of it, really. Okay, the doctor told us what it is but you just keep thinking: 'Oh, goodness me, what if they forget her? What if they forget her in a corner somewhere or out in the corridor?' I'd die. It really makes you worried when it's happened before, and from the time she fell and broke her hip it's been bad all the way.

It doesn't really get any better, and you just worry. I may take the day off the first time she goes; I won't go with her because the ambulance picks lots of people up. She won't want me sitting in a hospital all day with her watching everything that goes on, either, but at least I can see her being taken off, and they can come in to get her.

It does worry me now this business with the day hospital; they tell you how the ambulance or the bus works, but you're not quite sure. I went with her in the ambulance once; that was a nightmare, but that's another story.

They picked up a few people on the way and they picked up this lady. I haven't got a clue what was wrong with her, but we stopped off to pick up another gentleman and the ambulance men went to help him, and this woman had some kind of muscle spasms and she couldn't control her movements at all. She took out of her bag this folder thing with a load of pills in it and they were all in their daily dosage. Of course she couldn't control what she was doing – she took them all out and they all went flying everywhere. I sat there thinking: 'Oh dear, what do I do? What do I do?' and they went all over the place. She was fidgeting all over them and picking them up and she started to put them in her mouth. I thought: 'I can't just sit and watch this,' so I took what I could off her and I picked up the rest from the floor and she was saying: 'Thank you, thank you.' They were everywhere and I was sitting there thinking: 'Oh my God, when are those men coming back? What do I do? What do I do?'

Mum was just sitting there, this was going on behind her – she can't see and she can't hear very well. I don't know how many tablets the woman had got in her mouth – she was trying to pick up more from the floor and I was trying to get them off the floor before she could. I was so glad when the ambulance men came back, and I just said: 'You know you've got a problem here,' and I left them and climbed into the front of the ambulance.

Getting out

It is difficult. I was saying to her that when the weather warms up, maybe we'll hire a wheelchair because she hasn't been out apart from her visits to the hospital. She was very active – she'd take a walk and go up to the shops and things like that. The other day she got up on her crutches and opened the front door just to breathe in a bit of fresh air.

There are places you can hire wheelchairs and things; they're very expensive to buy; we'll get her out a bit into the fresh air, silly things like that. I'm sure to Mum it's a wonderful thought for her to be able to go out again.

She was getting on okay at the day hospital and she went to the hairdressers on her own, which was a bit scary, then the next time she went back to the day hospital she fell over. She didn't do any damage, but obviously she got a bit frightened after that. She's been back to the hairdressers, actually, but with somebody.

INDEX

Page references in *italics* indicate figures or tables